Goerner

the Mighty

By Edgar Mueller

DISCLAIMER

The exercises and advice contained within this book is for educational and entertainment purposes only. The exercises described may be too strenuous or dangerous for some people, and the reader should consult with a physician before engaging in any of them.

The author and publisher of this book are not responsible in any manner whatsoever for any injury, which may occur through the use or misuse of the information presented here.

Goerner the Mighty originally published in 1951

Modern Reprint Edition
Copyright © 2012 by StrongmanBooks.com
All Rights Reserved.

No part of this course may be reproduced or transmitted in any form or by any means, electronic or mechanical, including photocopying, recording, or by any information storage and retrieval system, without permission in writing from the publisher.

Manufactured in the United States of America

GOERNER
The Mighty

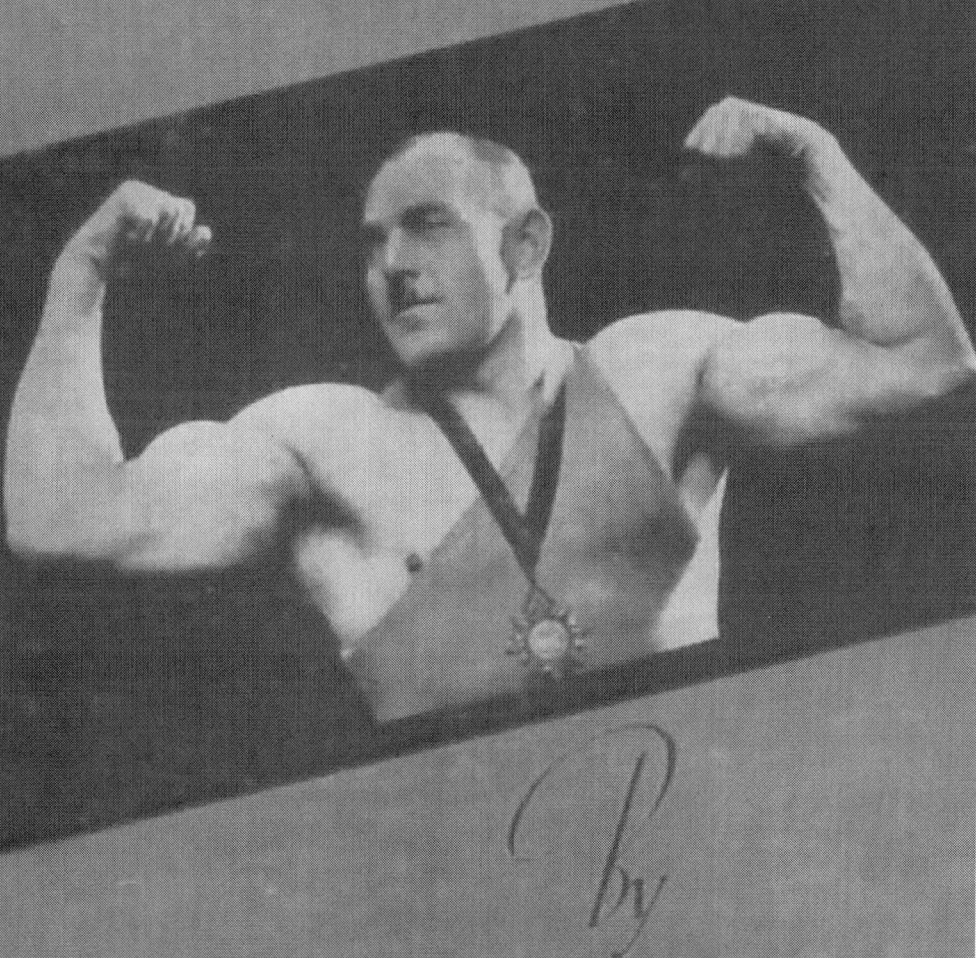

By
EDGAR MUELLER

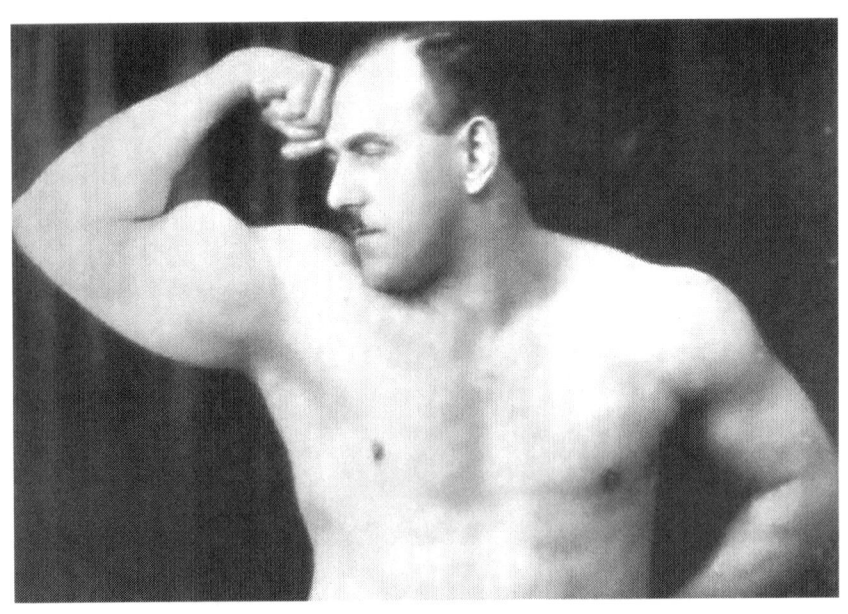

Hermann Görner – age 30

Biceps, 19 in. Chest, 54 in. Neck, 10 ½ in. Weight, 260 lb.

CONTENTS

		PAGE
Foreword.	Irving R. Clark	5
Introduction.	John E. Dawe	9
Chapter 1.	Introduction Hermann Görner	12
Chapter 2.	His Early Life	16
Chapter 3.	His Later Life and Travels	26
Chapter 4.	His Measurements	32
Chapter 5.	His Lifting Performances and Feats of Strength	36
Chapter 6.	His Training Methods	68
Chapter 7.	His Attitude to Strength Feats	94
Conclusion.	Appreciation – by World Famous Authorities	105

ILLUSTRATIONS

Hermann Görner	Frontispiece
Wrestling with an Elephant	11
Carrying Four Men on One Shoulder	14
Görner at 36 Years of Age	18
The Hermann Strongfort Trio	20
Two Hands Jerk with Live Weights	24
The Human Bridge	28
Supporting a Ballet Company	31
Finish of the Ballet Company's Act	35
Hermann Görner (posed)	39
Hermann Görner at age 43	43
Hermann and Elsie Görner	45
A Corner of Edgar Müller's Gymnasium	49
Hermann Görner at age 17	52
Another Pose of Görner at 17 years	53
Hermann Görner – age 18 years	56
Hermann Görner with Karl Swoboda	60
Hermann Görner with Otto Brauer	63
Edgar Müller in his Gymnasium	66
Görner Training in the open air	70
Hermann Görner lifting his "Challenge" barbell	73
Lifting 595 ¾ lbs. with Four Fingers	77
Hermann Görner doing the "Plank" feat	80
Sketch showing measurements of brick	82
Sketch – Lifting 10 bricks with one hand	83
Pinch-grip lifting 111 lbs. with one hand	86
Stacking 32 bricks at once	91
One way of lifting 14 bricks at once	95
Snatching a barbell in an unusual manner	101
One handed weight throwing	104
Two Hands pinch-grip Snatch – Style A	108
Two Hands pinch-grip Snatch – Style B	109

To My Friend

HERMANN GÖRNER

"The Strongest Man Who Ever Lived"

FOREWORD

"The good old days" is a by-word. Most times the operative word is "old", and distance lends its enchantment, but when one turns to the professional weight lifting sphere one is also entitled to refer to the "good not-so-old days".

For the decade ending as recently as 1930 threw up many great Strong Men, perhaps not as eccentric in their hair-cuts nor skirted like Cyr, not as beautiful as Sandow, nor as bombastic as Sampson; unframed by gilt and plush, but displaying feats of strength sometimes even more laudable than those of their illustrious predecessors, if with simpler instruments and in a different manner.

Like their comrades of the 90's, they were a cosmopolitan crowd. The Russian Zass, the Pole Breitbart, the Frenchmen Cadine and Rigoulot, and the German Görner . . . . And the greatest of these, I think, was Görner.

Cast in a gigantic mould; one seldom used for Strong Men, almost that of the old time Austrian Türk and the French Uni, (Apollon) his over 6 ft. of height was underpinned by 17½ st. of smooth proportionate muscle.

Interest in the professional scene having been recreated by two matches in 1925 and 1926 for the title of World's Strongest Man, contested by the two Frenchman and both won by Charles Rigoulot, I shall never forget the excitement caused by Tromp van Diggelen's publication of some articles about an "unknown" (see later) who could lift nearly 800 lb. off the ground, wrestle with a baby elephant, take the weight of a laden motor-car upon his shoulders, and perform other feats of the superhuman variety.

This, of course, was Görner, and he and his wife, almost as strong as he in supporting feats, duly arrived in England in 1927, and under the aegis of W.A. Pullum gave some proof of his immense strength by Dead Lifting before British Officials, in strict British styles, rulings and on appliances strange to him, over 650 lb. with two hands and 600 lb. with one, together with a number of other feats . . . and then seemed to fade out of the picture. I say 'seemed', and I called him an 'unknown' in the last paragraph, rather in the style of our headline about the Channel gale which Europeans use to illustrate our insularity: 'High Seas in English Channel. Shipping at a Standstill. Continent Isolated'.

Rigoulot, on the other hand, went on from strength to strength to make the 'impossible' grades of an over 250 lb. one hand Snatch, an over 300 lb. two hands ditto and an over 400 lb. Clean and Jerk. Unfortunately, the two, Görner and Rigoulot, never met. (Or did they? Wild horses will not drag from Görner some little stories about this). The stumbling block was that the German, not unnaturally, would have played his two or three trump cards, the Dead Lifts; spelling curtains for the Frenchman. That, of course, is conjecture at best. What Müller has written in this volume appears to me to be reality.

I have met both Hermann and his biographer, Edgar Müller, in their native land, where they both live in straitened circumstances as flüchtlinge (refugees), far from their homes. Despite the loss of his wife and his fortune, and his 16 months in a Concentration Camp including work in a mine, Hermann is still the genial figure, with an eye to a joke, who endeared himself to British audiences in 1927. Apart from a small pension (he lost an eye in the first World War), he has practically nothing left except the clothes he stands up in, the bedding he sleeps in, some bills and hand-outs from Pagel's Circus with which he featured in South Africa many times, and an article I wrote about him in *Superman* about 15 years ago.

A word also about Edgar Müller, who is almost unknown to British readers. 'If Edgar says it is so, it is so', should be the slogan over the Müller portal. I pride myself on being a judge of precise, exact, factual people and I have never met such a walking encyclopedia on continental Strong Men and their feats, as this man. Mention a feat and he can state the date, the time, who was present; almost the state of the weather and 'the colour of the engine driver's tie'.

He is a sheer 'fanatic' on weight lifting and weight training and can discourse for hours, days if necessary, both in his native German and in very good English, on the subject. Since 1943, when nearly the whole of his cuttings, records, photographs, books and charts were destroyed by fire, he has slowly built up a small but comprehensive indexed record of feats and personalities. It is not only from this that you get this story; its authenticity is copper-bottomed by his close friendship and co-operation with Herman Görner over 30 years; the whole cemented by his amazing memory.

To test some of his statements, I made a few enquiries myself about Görner's amazing two hands Dead Lift of nearly 800 lb. I pointed out to Edgar that whilst 'Brockhaus', the German equivalent of the *Encyclopedia Britannica*, accepted this lift in its 1922 edition as authentic, Theodor Siebert, the great German trainer of Weight Lifters and sometimes Stronger Men, gave the big man credit for only 300 kg. in a book he published in 1923. Quick as a flash, Edgar referred me to a German magazine of 1926 (which I had missed) in which Siebert acknowledges the greater feat.

There was another little matter, too, which illustrates his card-index recollection. In two American magazines in the 1940's mention was made of a German, Paul Whur, alleged to have been the first man in the world to Clean and Jerk the double bodyweight. At least that was to me the inference from the date 1904. Astounding because the first previous recorded instances were at the Olympic Games of 1928. A little matter of 24 hours can sometimes make a difference in the weight lifting world . . . but 24 *years*!

So I duly consulted the oracle and his reply was that there was a *Joseph Wühr* round about that time, who was *Continental-Jerking* (a far different proposition) weights approaching the double bodyweight. (He gave me the figures from his records. Actually, one of the magazines in question changed its mind about the feat and eventually called it a Continental Jerk).

Just now, I couldn't care less whether or not Wühr lifted the double bodyweight overhead. What I am interested in is Accuracy, and I think the reading public is too. That is why I commend this book,

www..StrongmanBooks.com

hoping it will be the forerunner of many.

IRVING CLARK,
Fully Qualified Referee of the
British Amateur Weightlifters' Association,
Formerly Honorary Legal Adviser to the
B.A.W.L.A.

INTRODUCTION

Introducing Edgar Müller

In presenting to the world of strength the first full and authentic life story of Hermann Görner, it is appropriate to introduce his biographer, Edgar Müller.

Writer, teacher, referee, statistician and historian, Edgar Müller is, without any doubt, the most knowledgeable authority on Weight Lifting, Strength Feats and Strong Men in Germany at the present time.

Born at Nossen, in Saxony, on 15th November, 1898, he served in the first World War and saw action in Belgium and France from 1917-1919, being discharged finally on account of war wounds.

He studied physical culture at the Institut für Leibesübungen der Universität, Leipzig (School of Physical Culture of Leipzig University). In business on his own account as a Fur Trader, he also established and managed one of the best known and most fully-equipped gymnasiums in Germany, situated in Leipzig. Due to air action, he lost his business and his home, together with much of his amazing collection of rare and unique books, cuttings, photographs and records of Weight Lifting, Strength Feats and Strong Men throughout the ages and from the world over.

In 1916 he won his first Junior Title in Weight Lifting and shortly after this found himself very impressed by the teachings and writings of Professor Theodor Siebert, after whose methods he modelled his own system of training to be put into effect in his gymnasium later. He was Secretary and Referee for the Athletic Club Samson, when only 21 years of age. In 1920 he met Hermann Görner for the first time and throughout the years to the present day their friendship has continued unbroken. In 1929, Edgar Müller suffered a severe accident in falling down an ice-covered stairway and badly injured bones in his left hand, which hindered him considerably in his weight lifting career. Nevertheless, he was lifting officially as recently as 1944, when he won the Championship of Saxony at Chemnitz, at the age of 46. In 1930, he was elected Weight Lifting Instructor, Judge and Team Coach to three Leipzig Clubs – namely, ' The Atlas ', 'Dala' and 'Arthur Saxon Weight Lifting Club', which duties he carried out over the period 1930-1937. During these years, he promoted and staged many Mr. Leipzig contests and Weight Lifting Meetings on the 'Olympic' and other Lifts.

In this same year (1930), he founded his own school in Leipzig, which catered for Weight Lifters, Body Builders and Strength Artises. He was also the principal founder of the 'Hermann Görner Club', Leipzig. In 1936 at the Berlin Olympic Games, he reported the Weight Lifting events for a Leipzig newspaper and on this occasion Edgar Müller met many of the world's best known figures of strength, including our own Heavyweight Champion at that time – the late Ronald Walker of Wakefield. It is of great interest to British readers to note that Edgar Müller has the greatest admiration for the feats of strength and amazing lifts established by Ronald Walker, whose career Edgar Müller always followed closely. It is Mr. Müller's considered opinion that Ronald Walker was the world's strongest man, at his weight, when in his lifting prime.

Edgar Müller has trained many of Saxony's champion lifters with his methods which he developed in conjunction with Hermann Görner.

In 1947, he left Leipzig (now in the Russian Zone) and came to reside in the British Zone, after closing down his gymnasium, which he had continued to operate. He has suffered severely through his experiences resulting from the aftermath of World War II, but his enthusiasm is still boundless. His ambition is to found an Anglo/German Weight Lifting Club in conjunction with Hermann Görner to be run on a cultural basis in the British Zone of Germany.

JOHN E. DAWE,

Fully Qualified Referee of the

British Amateur Weight Lifters Association.

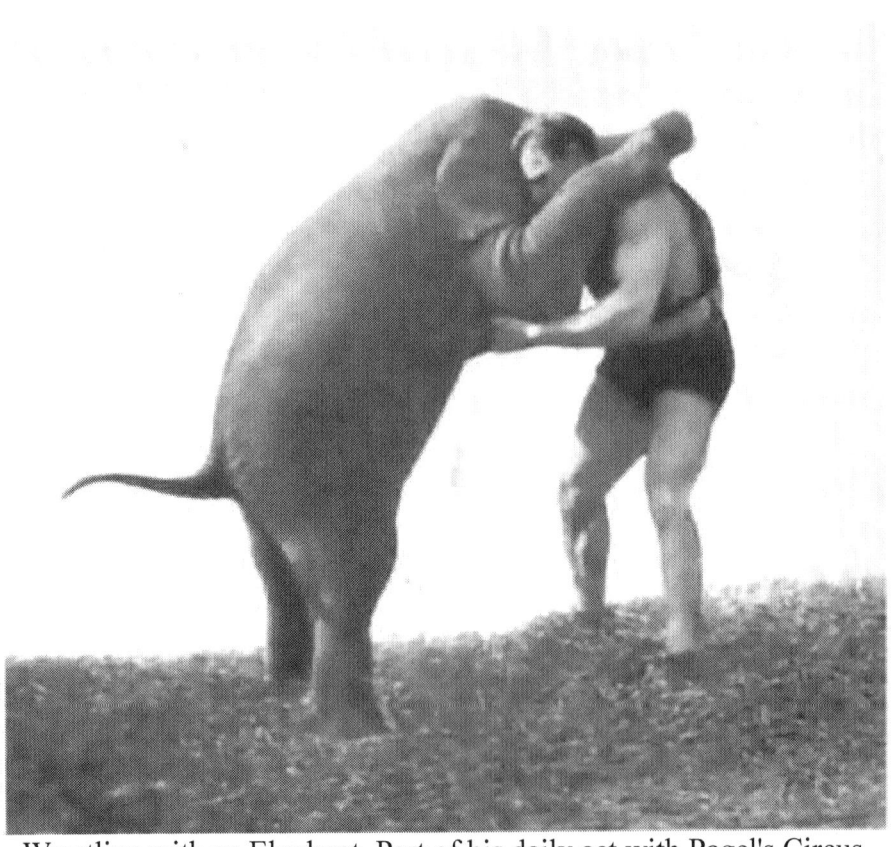

Wrestling with an Elephant. Part of his daily act with Pagel's Circus, South Africa. The elephant weighed 700 lb. at the comencement of the tour and had increased to 1500 lb. by the end of the tour, but was handled just as easily by the mighty Görner.

EDGAR MÜLLER

GOERNER THE MIGHTY

By Edgar Müller

CHAPTER I

Introducing Hermann Görner

BEFORE I met Hermann Görner, I had so often read of his name in connection with extraordinary feats of physical power that the desire to meet him became an obsession with me.

My chance came in 1920 and the first glimpse I had of this towering superman gave me a feeling of overwhelming awe – I had seen other physical giants, including the Russian mastodon, Feodor Machnow, who stood 8 ft. 9 ½ in. and weighed about 34 stones; I have met Primo Carnera, when he came to Leipzig in 1929, but none gave me the thrill that I experienced as I gazed for the first time on our friend – the smiling, unflurried Hermann Görner with a figure truly Herculean yet not without an easy grace.

Görner's six feet of manhood is almost dwarfed by the extraordinary spread of shoulder he possesses. He is a man of huge symmetrical bulk without any vestige of adiposity. The huge masses of muscle on his arms, back and legs were to me something out of this world. Never had I seen such a figure – never had I been so impressed and to this day this impression has survived.

After the theatre had closed on his performances, he would discard his leotard and don his street attire. You could not mistake him, even if one covered him with a shroud. He was still a magnificent figure walking leisurely along the street. Clothes, no matter how well tailored they might be, betrayed the startling evidence of thews rippling under protesting cloth. His neck was like that of a young bull and made his collar appear inadequate. Hands and wrists that gave every indication of a vice-like grip; a stride and manner that vibrated glorious strength in every step – here was the living incarnation of what we had been led to believe existed in the past, when they paid tribute to man's physical superiority in statutes of bronze and marble.

On meeting Hermann for the first time, I was surprised to notice that his voice and manner of speaking was startingly quiet. Modest and gentle, but the twinkle in his eye indicated he was not averse to a sense of good humour and as I became better acquainted with him, I discovered he was also very fond of what the British call 'leg pulling', but always without a hint of malice, being nothing less than sheer exuberance that is not unusual with men so gifted with abundant strength and bubbling heath.

I was, however, to discover that my friend did not possess a one-track mind personality. Hermann could express himself delightfully on the piano and accordion. A game of chess or a game of billiards would often fill a spare hour in between performances.

A quiet man, a peace-loving man; honouring that which is right, detesting that which is wrong; a healthy abhorrence of regimentation and all that it might imply; deploring the causes that make men forget, so that in their militaristic amnesia they destroy with legal impunity what Nature created to be the most perfect physical machine in a world of moving things.

A respector of his fellow men, gallant to the weaker sex and those not so blessed with physical qualifications; a philosopher who had learned that the trials and stresses of life visit both the strong and the weak.

Elsie Görner, Hermann's wife, a lady of bearing serious and of great understanding, bade her adieu to this world early in 1949. This sad blow to Hermann left him bereft of his staunchest champion. This shock coming after a period that had left the world wounded and trying to regain its balance after the human catastrophe, which had been shared by all, might have bowed lesser men than Görner, but he was of sterner mettle. Hermann Görner was not just strong in physical power – he had the mental qualifications which resist and repel attacks on the less obvious senses – a great body and a great mind were in harmony.

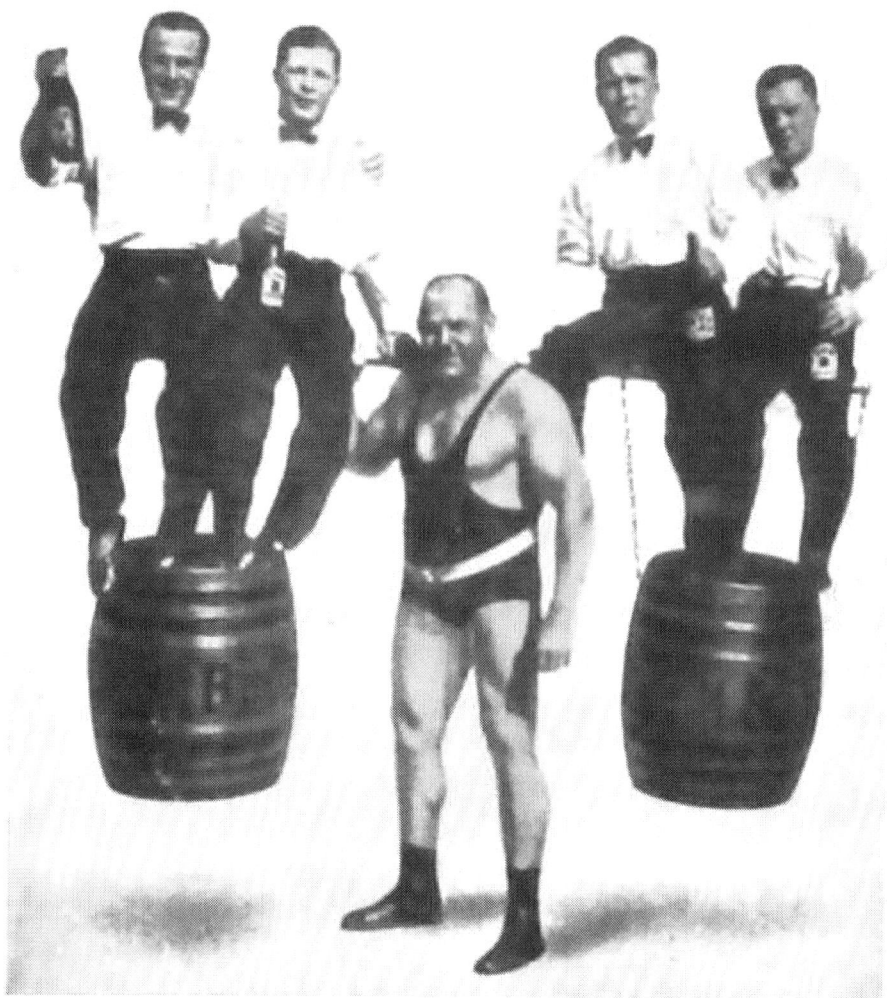

Carrying four men on one shoulder – total weight over 1000 lb. Performed in South Africa as part of his circus act in his 1935 tour.

Shocks might shake and temporarily flounder most of us but with time and understanding the strong survive even the most severe catastrophies.

Elsie Görner, during her life, which had been devoted to Hermann, had made a hobby of collecting and preserving anything literary referring to her husband – press reports, magazine cuttings, excerpts, articles, announcements, tributes coming from every corner of the world. She was justly proud of her world adulated man. When things were normal, his good wife had learned that, to keep Hermann in the pink of condition, he needed sufficient sleep, as much as 4 ½ lb. of minced meat with eggs thrown in to help along. He has always been a moderate drinker and smoker.

To-day Hermann Görner lives alone in a tiny village not far from Hannover in Germany. His home is nothing more than a small room in which he eats, sleeps, cooks and philosophies. It contains a bed, a table, two chairs, a cupboard and a small stove for heating and cooking purposes. A far cry from the comfortable home he once had in Leipzig and vastly different also from the prosperous restaurant he once managed and lived in. In his present one-roomed 'home' Hermann often receives interviews with transient followers of the cult of strength. Here in this tiny home, the author has spent many a long hour talking, discussing and reviewing practically everything men do in similar circumstances, especially when a common bond exists between them.

CHAPTER 2

His Early Life

HERMANN GÖRNER was born in Haenichen near Leipzig on 13th April, 1891. He was the youngest of three children and at birth showed nothing unusual to indicate the great power that was later to be his. In fact, he weighed so little that it was thought he would never amount to very much physically. However, by the time he was three years of age, young Hermann grew to normal size for a child of this age. His father was a big-boned giant standing nearly 6 ft. 3 in. in height, but his mother was little over 5 ft. tall. His father wore on his small finger a ring which Hermann could wear with ease on his thumb and this was many years later, when Hermann was a full-grown man.

In spite of the pessimistic predictions at his birth, Hermann grew up into a fine, sturdy boy, showing excellent bone and muscular possibilities. At 10 years of age, he became interested in Weight Lifting. At the age of 14 – his last term at school – he was able to swing to full stretch of the arm a kettleweight weighing 110 ¼ lb. (50 kilos). At this time he stood 5 ft. 6 1/8 in. (168 cms.) and weighed 185 ¼ lb. (84 kilos) or 13 stone 3¼ lb. As a matter of interest, George Hackenschmidt, the famous 'Russian Lion' was said to have been 4 ft. 7½ in. in height and 122 lb. or 8 stone 10 lb. in weight at the same age, according to his book, 'The Way to Live'.

It is interesting to note that, contrary to popular belief, Hermann's practice of Weight Lifting at the early age of 10 years did not have the effect of preventing his later growth to a height of 6 ft. 0½in. (184 cms.). In this connection, also, it may be mentioned that another famous strong man, Louis Uni of France, better known as Apollon, started the practice of Weight Lifting at the age of 12 and reached the height of 6 ft. 3 in. at maturity (1.90 cms.).

It is worthy of note that all famous strong men have served an apprenticeship at outdoor sports in the course of which they have laid the foundation of their vigorous 'animal' strength, vitality and health.

Hermann Görner is no exception to this. He practised all manner of health-giving outdoor sports – running, jumping, swimming, acrobatics, shot and weight putting in addition to boxing and wrestling.

It was apparent that as he grew and developed his musculature retained its sharp clearly defined lines. At 18 years of age he had attained measurements worthy of a full-grown strong man. His biceps, neck and calves were each 17 in. (Exactly 43 cms.) in circumstance. His trade of Stove Fitter, however, gave Hermann little scope for his growing talents.

Famous sculptors, including Professor Klinger and Professor Moutier, were enraptured over his physique. He was engaged by them to pose for many of their works and, through this and other means, Hermann soon discovered that there were many ways of adding to his income whenever he felt like exhibiting his tremendous physique and great strength.

By the time he was 21 years old, Hermann had won many honours in Weight Lifting including the following successes: –

Championship of Middle Germany, 1911.
Championship of Brandenburg Province, 1911.
Championship of Northern Germany, 1911.
Second in Championship of Europe, 1911.
Second in Championship of Middle Germany, 1912.
Winner of National Contest in Berlin, 1912.

During the years 1911-13, Hermann Görner was the leader of a Strong Man Trio. The Trio was first known as the 'Atlas Trio', later the title was changed to the 'Hermann Strongfort Trio', the members consisting of Hermann himself, his brother, Otto Görner and a friend, Otto Brauer. The Trio – all amateurs – put over an excellent act, featuring numbers in which they worked together intermixed with solo numbers. The act was opened with simultaneous juggling of kettleweights by the Trio, this being followed by juggling with a Globe barbell. Next the stage was taken by Hermann Görner as the featured

EDGAR MÜLLER

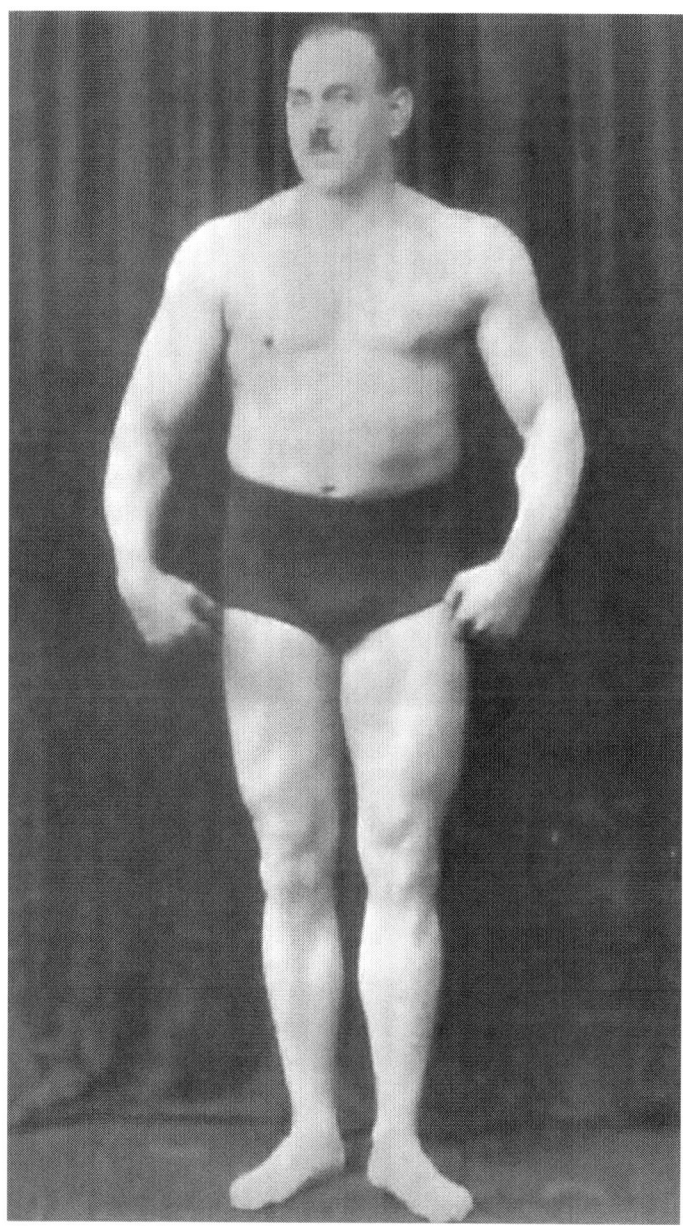

Görner at 36 years of age. A relaxed pose showing his symmetrical development. Photograph taken during his stay in England in 1928.

performer. Taking a specially-constructed bar at either end of which one of his partners sat, he would jerk the whole overhead with two hands – the Jerk being made from behind the neck. This feat was then followed by Otto Brauer bent pressing with the right hand a kettleweight on which a man was seated, following up the Bent Press by taking up from the floor and pressing overhead a second kettleweight. The next feat was carried out by Otto Görner. He supported across his shoulders a barbell and five men. One of the men was seated on his shoulders and two men were suspended from each end of the bar. When the whole load was in position, Otto then revolved rapidly several times on his own axis, finally returning the men and the barbell to the stage. The next number featured Hermann, this time supporting on his feet and hands in the pyramid position two barbells and eight men, the whole load being supported for several seconds. The concluding feature of the 'Hermann Strongfort Trio' was carried out by all three performers working together. The two Otto's laid on their backs and supported with their legs a stout plank, upon which eighteen or more men were placed, the men being lifted into position like babies by the redoubtable Hermann. As has been already said, this act was performed by the same trio for over two years, being performed in most of the principal cities of Middle Germany.

During 1922, Hermann again joined forces for a short time in a duo act with Otto Brauer. This time the act consisted of some ten different feats, performed singly and together, and including juggling with kettleweights and barbells, twirling a barbell around the body in the so-called 'Russian Mill' style. Hermann himself featured his famous challenge barbell with a shaft of 2 3/8 in. diameter and weight of 330 ¾ lb., which he cleaned and jerked overhead, then dropped to behind his neck, from which position it was again jerked overhead and finally dropped from arms length and caught in the crook of his arms, before replacing on the floor. The remaining features of the act included supporting a barbell and five men on the shoulders and whirling around, jerking overhead two men on a bar from behind the neck, supporting on a specially-built apparatus mounted on his head two men, who were then twirled around as if on a roundabout. This latter feature of the act was performed by Otto Brauer. Hermann featured a number

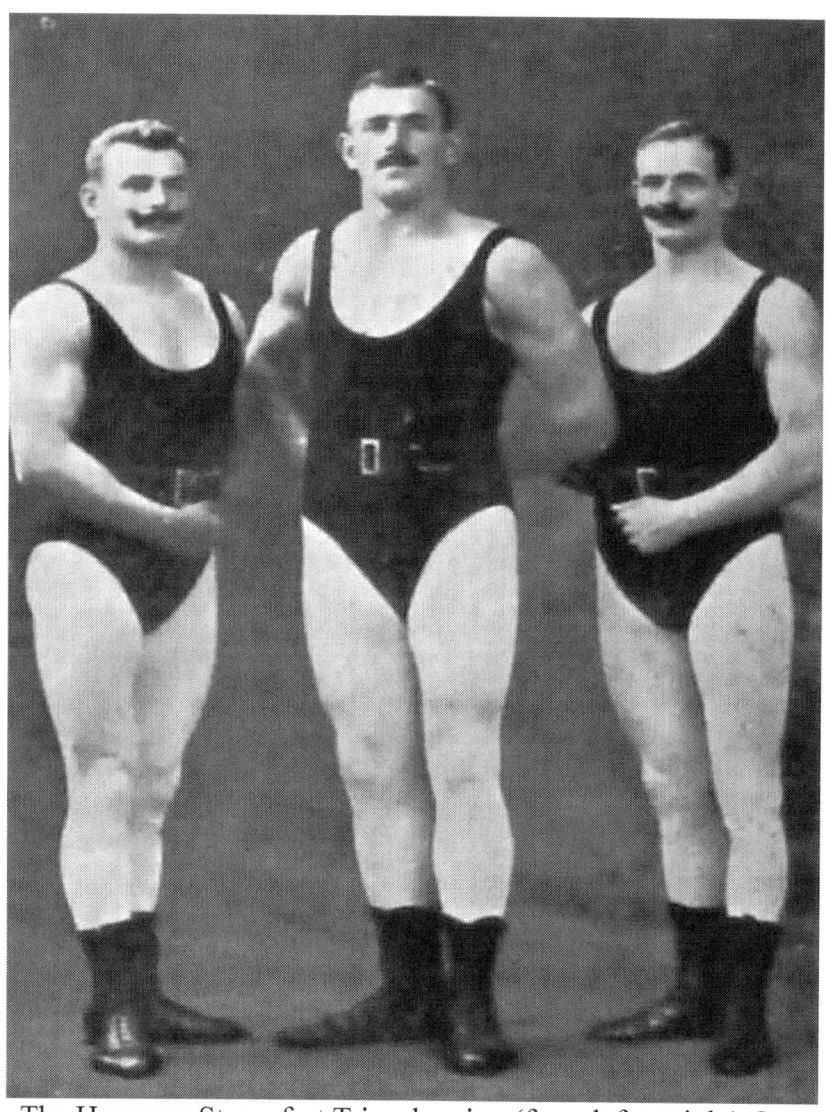

The Hermann Strongfort Trio, showing (from left to right) Otto Görner (Hermann's brother), Hermann Görner and Otto Brauer. Taken in Leipzig in 1911.

in which he danced a waltz around the stage, at the same time supporting on his right shoulder a barbell to which four men clung. Otto Brauer took the next feature of the act by lying on his back and supporting five men and two barbells, one of the men holding two kettleweights overhead – similar to the famous Roman Column. The final number of the act featured Hermann reclining on his back and supporting on his legs a revolving Merry-Go-Round on which eight men had a ride.

At the age of 22, Hermann lifted in the 1913 German Weight Lifting Championships at Kassel. In these Championships he was third in the Heavyweight Class, behind Paul Trappen of Trier and Karl Mörke of Koeln (Cologne). This Championship was decided on 5 Lifts, namely, One Arm Snatch, One Arm Jerk, Two Hands Press, Two Hands Snatch and Two Hands Clean and Jerk. Görner lifted a total of 1,146 lb. (520 kilos) against Trappen's winning total of 1,217 ½ lb. (552 ½ kilos) and Mörke's 1,212 lb. (550 kilos) which gave him second place. Hermann's individual Lifts were: –

One Hand Snatch	170 ¾ lb. (77 ½ kilos).
One Hand Jerk	203 ¾ lb. (92 ½ kilos).
Two Hands Snatch	231 ¼ lb. (105 kilos).
Two Hands Press	220 ½ lb. (100 kilos).
Two Hands Clean and Jerk	319 ½ lb. (145 kilos).

In 1913 Hermann Görner also lifted in the World's Championships held in Breslau on 26th to 28th July of that year, but due to his having to work more than ten hours per day at this particular period he was not able to find sufficient time to train properly, so could not reproduce his best form. He finished fourth, behind Josef Grafl of Vienna, who won with a total of 975 lb. on the four lifts of Right Hand Snatch, Left Hand Snatch, Two Hands Press and Two Hands Continental Jerk with Barbell. Berthold Tandler of Vienna was second and Jan Krausse of Riga, third.

Although it may now seem strange, in the light of what has happened, Hermann WANTED to be a boxer or wrestler, but these plans were shattered by the 1914/18 war and after serving four years

EDGAR MÜLLER

'Dienst bei der Fahne' – Service with the Colours – he returned home having sustained severe shrapnel wounds and being blind in both eyes. He later underwent a very delicate operation by a famous eye specialist and sight was restored to his left eye, but the other was totally destroyed. Notwithstanding this heavy setback his fighting heart was undaunted and he made plans for the future which he proceeded to put into immediate operation.

Hermann recommenced training as soon as he was reasonably fit and entered his name for the 1919 German Weight Lifting Championships which were held in that year in München (Munich) on 9th and 10th August. On this occasion, the famous Karl Mörke emerged the winner with Hermann Görner runner-up. The Lifts were the same five Lifts as in 1913 but due to the intervention of the war years and lack of training facilities, the totals registered were appreciably lower than in 1913. Mörke totalled 1,190 lb. (540 kilos) against Görner's 1,124 lb. (510 kilos) with the celebrated Josef Strassberger third with 1,107 ¼ lb. (502 ½ kilos). Up to this time it is interesting to note that Hermann was still an amateur Weight Lifter.

In 1920 The World Championships were held in Vienna, the winner in the Heavyweight Class being Karl Mörke, beating Aigner and Alscher, both of Austria, into second and third places. Mörke's winning lifts were Right Hand Snatch 165 ¼ lb. (75 kilos), Right Hand Jerk (two hands to shoulder) 220 ½ lb. (100 kilos), Two Hands Press 242 ½ lb. (110 kilos), Two Hands Continental Jerk 350 lb. (162 ½ kilos). In this year, 1920, a match was arranged between Karl Mörke and Hermann Görner. Hermann was out to avenge his defeat by Mörke in 1919 German Weight Lifting Championships.

The match was a battle between the 'long and the short of it' – as a note about the men's respective physiques will reveal. Hermann standing over six feet in height and Karl Mörke barely five feet, two-and-a-half inches, weighing 220 lb., and nearly as broad as he was tall!

The match duly took place on 4th April, 1920, in the Restaurant Hall of the Zoological Gardens, Leipzig, and was held on the following Lifts: –

GOERNER THE MIGHTY

> One Hand Snatch.
> One Hand Jerk.
> Two Hands Press.
> Two Hands Snatch.
> Two Hands Jerk.

The sixth Lift being a Lift selected by each man. This was in Hermann's case the Two Hands Dead Lift and, in Karl Mörke's case, the Deep Knee Bend. The result of this Match, refereed by Paul Schröder, was a decisive win for Hermann Görner, as the following details will show: –

	HERMANN GÖRNER	KARL MÖRKE
	Right-hand Snatch	*Right-hand Snatch*
	198 ¼ lb. (90 kilos)	165 ½ lb. (75 kilos)
	Right-hand Jerk	*Right-hand Jerk*
	248 lb. (112 ½ kilos) (Clean)	220 ¼ lb. (100 kilos) (Two hands to shoulder)
	Two-hands Press	*Two-hands Press*
	242 ½ lb. (110 kilos)	264 ½ lb. (120 kilos)
	Two-hands Snatch	*Two-hands Snatch*
	275 ½ lb. (125 kilos)	242 ½ lb. (110 kilos)
	Two-hands Jerk	*Two-hands Jerk*
	352 ½ lb. (160 kilos) (Clean)	341 ½ lb. (155 kilos) (Continental)
Totals	1,316 ¾ lb. (597 ½ kilos)	1,234 ¼ lb. (560 kilos)
	Two-hands Dead Lift	*Deep Knee Bend*
	661 lb. (300 kilos)	528 ¾ lb. (240 kilos)
Grand Totals	1,977 ¾ lb. (897 ½ kilos)	1,763 lb. (800 kilos)

EDGAR MÜLLER

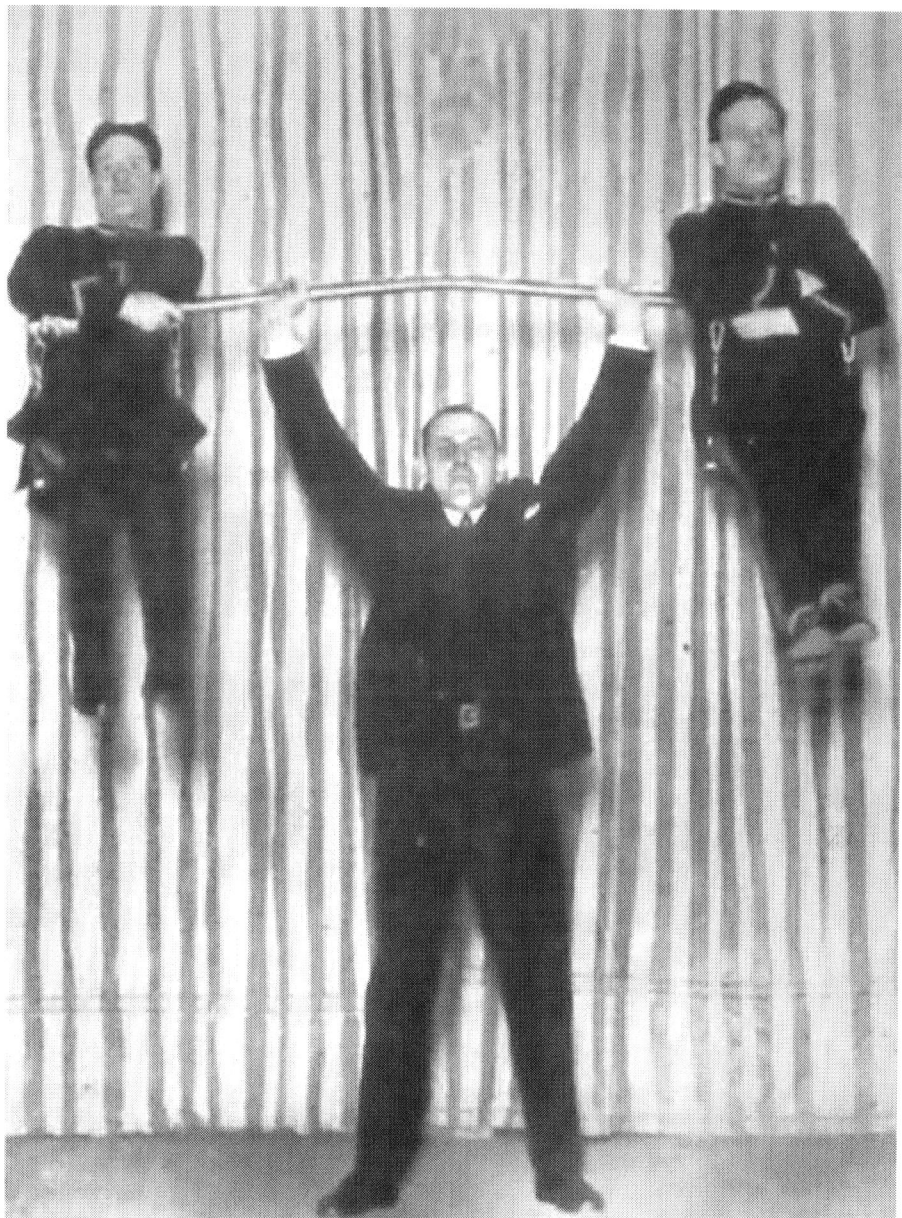

Two-hands Jerk with live weights – totalling 392 lb. Photograph taken in England in 1927.

It will thus be seen that Hermann decisively beat the World's Champion Heavyweight Weight Lifter and by his powerful lifting clearly demonstrated that he was not as his best form the previous year, when Mörke emerged the winner against Hermann in the Championships held in Munich.

Karl Mörke later went to America, where he resided for some years. He later returned to Germany and died there in 1947 as a result, it is said, of injuries sustained in a bombing raid during the closing stages of World War II.

CHAPTER 3

His Later Life and Travels

In 1921 Hermann Görner became a professional Strong Man. Having become the 'World's Strongest Amateur Weight Lifter' in the Heavyweight Class, by his defeat of Karl Mörke, the World's Champion, Hermann turned to the ranks of Professional Strong Men and Strength Artistes, as a means of livelihood at which he could earn an income far in excess of that which would be his by following his former trade of stove fitter.

In 1922, on 27th May to be precise, Hermann was married in Berlin and with his wife set sail for South Africa on 29th June of that year. Until early 1924, Hermann and Elsie Görner travelled South Africa with the well-known Pagel's Circus, featuring a star act presenting artistically feats of strength of a magnitude never before seen even in that Continent famed for its men of strength.

Hermann's act included supporting on his shoulders one side of a bridge, whilst a fully laden motor-car was driven across. This breathtaking feat is fully described in Chapter 7. Other items in his act were: –

> Carrying and walking with 4 men sustained by a bar carried on his right shoulder.

> Juggling with kettleweights weighing 110¼ lb. (50 kilos) each.

> Lifting his stage barbell weighing 330¾ lb. (150 kilos) with a shaft of 2 3/8 in. diameter in the Two Hands Clean and Jerk style. This was his challenge barbell – it was never once lifted correctly by any challenger during all his tours of South Africa.

> Supporting a Merry-Go-Round on his feet, whilst lying on his back. In this feat, eight men were seated on the roundabout and whirled round merrily for several minutes.

GOERNER THE MIGHTY

The 'plank' feat with sixteen or more men sitting on a plank, supported by Görner's mighty legs, was also featured by him in his act.

Hermann made, in all, five tours of South Africa during the years 1922-1924, 1924-26, 1929-31, 1935-36 and, finally, 1937-38. His act was constantly varied and enlarged. One of his most sensational feats being his 'wrestling with an elephant' turn. This he performed daily – the elephant getting heavier as the days went by, until Hermann was finally handling no less than 1,500 lb. (680.4 kilos) of elephant – some wrestling partner!

Hermann has often told me that the weight of the beast did not worry him unduly, but the roughness of his hide did. It used to leave Hermann almost raw about the neck and shoulders after their daily tussle in the arena.

Hermann Görner was helped along the road to success as a Professional Strong Man and Circus Artiste in no small measure by the renowned Tromp van Diggelen of Capetown, South Africa. A few words about this man, who was instrumental later in introducing Hermann to W.A. Pullum of London, will not be out of place.

Tromp van Diggelen was born 1885 in Orange Free State, South Africa. He is by profession an engineer. In 1909 'Tromp' was the discoverer of the great Bavarian Strong Man and muscle-control expert, Max Sick later to be better known as Maxick. Tromp van Diggelen brought Maxick to England and subsequently piloted him to world-renowned fame. Maxick was the pioneer of 'muscle control' and a weight lifter of amazing ability.

Van Diggelen was, in his younger days, a Strong Man of repute himself. He is a teacher of Physical Culture and has written many valuable contributions to the literature of Physical Culture. In 1948 he flew to England to witness the Olympic Games held in London. He also acted as one of the judges for the 'Mr. Universe' competition, won by the famous John C. Grimek of U.S.A.

Hermann Görner would be the first to admit that he owes much

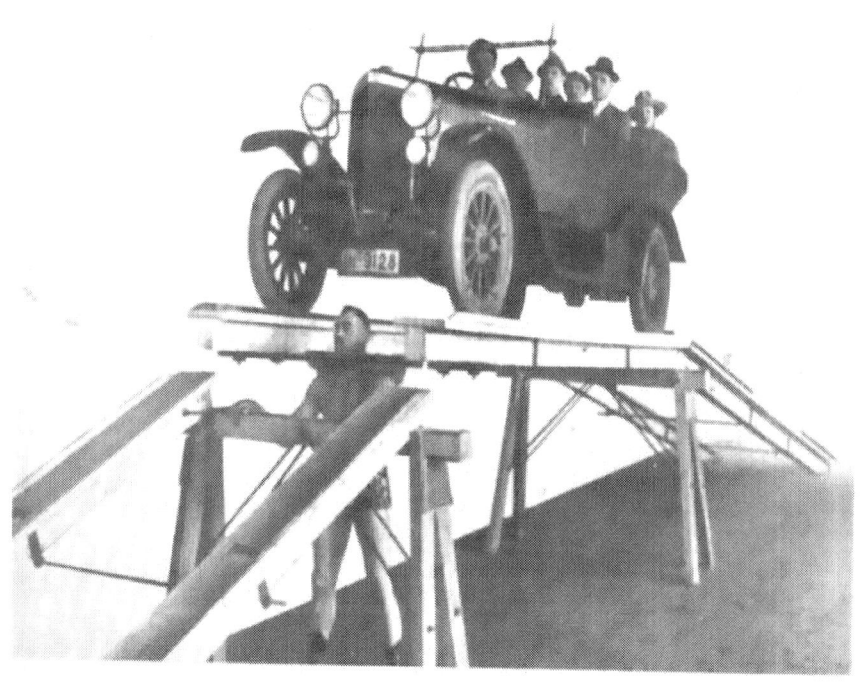

The Human Bridge – Hermann Görner supporting nearly 4000 lb. on his shoulders!

of his success and popularity to the mentor of his early days – Tromp van Diggelen.

In 1927/28 Görner was introduced to an amazed and admiring British public through the medium of W.A. Pullum – the 'Wizard of the Weights' of London. Pullum, for the benefit of those readers who may be unfamiliar with his career, was the former 9 stone (126 lb. – 57 kilos) Amateur Weight Lifting Champion of the World. He won over 50 gold medals and created close on 200 World and British Weight Lifting Records during his highly successful career as a lifter. Founder and Principal of the Camberwell Weight Lifting Club, he has trained, coached and managed scores of famous Strong Men. In 1948 W.A. Pullum was official coach to the British Olympic Weight Lifting Team, the members of which gained for Britain for the first time two Olympic medals for weight lifting. This, briefly, was the man introduced Görner to the British public. Hermann, in addition to Music Hall feats, established many amazing lifts during his stay in England – these are referred to in Chapter 7. Of Hermann's Music Hall act it may be mentioned that he incorporated the 'plank' feat made famous by Arthur Saxon. Hermann performed this feat nightly both in England and South Africa, supporting regularly sixteen men – he never bothered what the men weighed and the weights so supported by him were anywhere between 2,500 and 3,000 pounds (1,114 to 1,361 kilos).

In his act, Hermann held up a platform upon his knees and chest upon which a company of six ballet dancers performed and the finale was with a company of no less than 12 adults – the whole lot being sustained by Hermann on occasions for as long as eight minutes at a stretch. Carrying on to the stage two huge suitcases, he would walk the full length of the stage, turn round and walk back to the centre. Then, lightly depositing his two suitcases, the sides would fall down and out stepped four chorus girls – two from each case!

Jerking a barbell overhead to which a man sat on either end was another spectacular feat of strength performed by Hermann. Whilst in England a short feature film of Hermann was made by a well-known Film Company. The film showed him displaying his physical prowess in many ways – running, jumping, posing and, of course, lifting weights.

This film showed him juggling with kettleweights and barbell, cleaning and jerking his famous challenge barbell of 330¾ lb., horseshoe and iron bar bending and breaking, in feats of agility jumping over chairs, etc., supporting a merry-go-round, doing the famous 'plank' feat and other stupendous feats of strength.

It should be stated that he was the only strength athlete in the world who, over a period of twenty years, could do at any time of the day or night, a Two Hands Clean and Jerk of 330 ¾ lb. on his Stage Barbell – without warming up! As has already been stated, this Barbell possessed a shaft of 2 3/8 in. in diameter, a fact which made this feat even more meritorious.

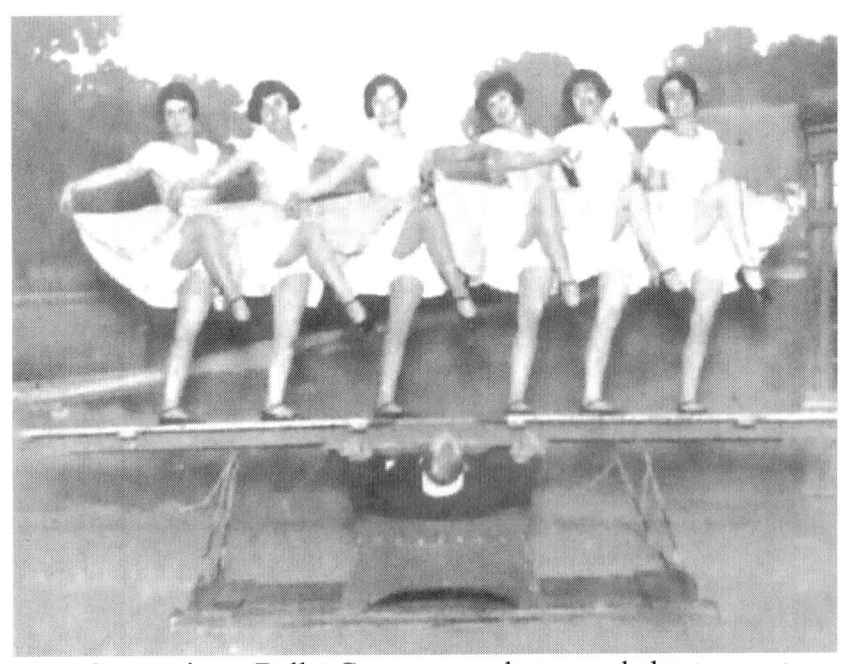
Supporting a Ballet Company on knees and chest as part of his Music Hall act.

CHAPTER 4

His Measurements

THE author took the following measurements of Hermann Görner on 16th December, 1934, when Hermann was 43 years of age. Weighing at this time 290 lb. or 20 stone 10 lb. (131 ½ kilos), he was about 30 lb. over his best lifting weight.

	Inches	*Centimeters*
Height	72.5	184
Neck	19.5	49.5
Reach (fingers tip to tip) – back against wall	78.3	199
Shoulder circumference, relaxed	59.1	150
Breadth of shoulders – normal	24	61
Chest – normal	50.4	128
Chest – expanded	54.4	138
Waist	45.25	115
Hips	46.5	118
Upperarm Straight – Right	17	43
Upperarm Straight – Left	16.2	41
Biceps – Right, flexed	18.9	48
Biceps – Left, flexed	18.1	46
Forearm Straight – Right	15.8	40
Forearm Straight – Left	15	38
Wrist – Right	9.1	23
Wrist – Left	8.7	22
Thigh – Right and Left	27.6	70
Knee – Right and Left	17.75	45
Calf – Right and Left	18.1	46
Ankle – Right and Left	11	28

These measurements were very carefully taken by myself and in all cases the tape was held horizontally and at right-angles to the bones and not slanted in any way to obtain an exaggerated measurement.

Anthropologists may be interested in the following additional measurements of Hermann, which have been taken from time to time by myself.

	Inches	Centimeters
Circumference of Head	22.9	58
Deltoid Circumference, with arm flexed at shoulder level – Right	23.25	59
Deltoid Circumference, with arm flexed at shoulder level – Left	22.1	56
Depth of chest – normal	12.6	32
Length of Hand	8.25	21
Breadth of Hand	4.4	11
Length of Foot – Right	11.8	30
Length of Foot – Left	12	30.5

He has a fresh complexion with medium blonde hair and blue eyes.

Due to his great width of shoulder, when one meets Hermann Görner in the flesh his height is not at first apparent and, indeed, from a distance one would imagine him to be of no more than average height or about 5 ft. 8 in. It is only when one is at close quarters with him that his tremendous bulk is fully appreciated.

Hermann's body weight at various periods in his life has been as follows: –

1905 – 185 ¼ lb. or 13 stone 3 ¼ lb.
1910 – 198 ½ lb. or 14 stone 2 ½ lb.
1913-1914 – 216 lb. or 15 stone 6 lb.
1919-1920 – 220 ½ lb. or 15 stone 10 ½ lb.
1925-1927 – 245 lb. or 17 stone 7 lb.
1929-1931 – 264 ½ lb. or 18 stone 12 ½ lb.
1934 – 290 lb. or 20 stone 10 lb.
1936-1939 – 293 ¼ lb. or 20 stone 13 ¼ lb.

His best maximum muscular weight at which he did many of his best performances, was 264 ½ lb. or 120 kilos.

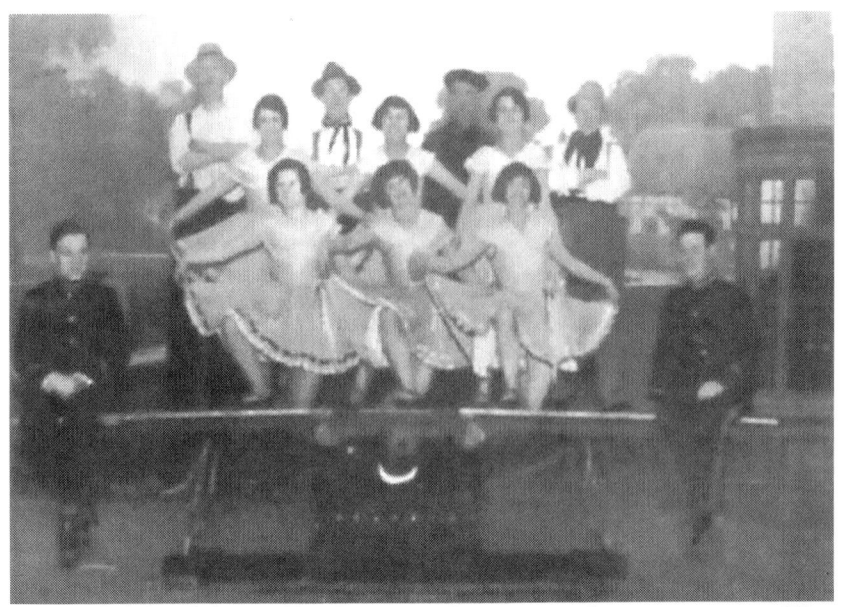

The finish of the Ballet Company's act – twelve persons totalling 2203 lb. – after an eight-minute performance – supported throughout by Hermann Görner.

EDGAR MÜLLER

CHAPTER 5

His Lifting Performances and Feats of Strength

I HAVE chosen to group the many wonderful feats performed during his career by Hermann Görner under headings classifying them into Single-Handed Lifts, Double-Handed Lifts and so on, rather than list them in strict chronological order. During the course of my association with Hermann, I have personally witnessed and recorded as a referee approximately 1,400 different feats of strength of all varieties and I have always had the impression that Hermann, in performing the greater majority of his many amazing feats, very rarely exerted himself to anywhere near the limits of his astounding power. In many cases, he could have exceeded the Lift he made at the time of performance by a further attempt, but this he always refused to do. Most of his established records were made with not more than two or three attempts. That he was undoubtedly one of the most accomplished all-round Strong Man and Weight Lifter the world has ever seen is my own firm conviction, and how correct or not is my judgment, I will leave to the reader, after he has carefully read the following list of some of the more outstanding of Görner's feats performed during the years I have been privileged to associate with him.

OVERHEAD LIFTS

Single-Handed Presses

Hermann has military pressed 137 ¾ lb. (62.5 kilos) with the right hand and 115 ¾ lb. (52.5 kilos) with the left hand. Arthur Saxon's best known military press, right hand, has been recorded at 126 lb. (57 kilos). Charles Rigoulot is said to have military pressed both right and left arm 119 lb. (54 kilos). Ronald Walker performed a right-hand military press of 128¾ lb. (58 ¼ kilos). The giant Swoboda military pressed with the right hand no less than 154¼ lb. (70 kilos) whilst Steinbach performed the same lift with 148¾ lb. (67.5 kilos). The best right-hand military press of Josef Grafl was 143¼ lb. (65 kilos).

Single-Handed Snatches

On 21st November, 1919, in Leipzig, Hermann snatched with the left hand 198½ lb. (90 kilos) and with the right hand he has snatched 229 ¼ lb. (104 kilos). This was on 4th September, 1926, when he had turned professional. Hermann's best lift as an amateur was 220 ½ lb. (100 kilos), lifted on 30th November, 1919, in Leipzig. The right-hand Snatch of Charles Rigoulot of 225 ¾ lb. (116 kilos) is the existing world's professional record. The best known Lift of Arthur Saxon was 200 lb. (91 kilos) on the right-hand Snatch, which was performed in 1900 in Leipzig. The famous British Heavy Weight Champion, Ronald Walker, had snatched with the right hand 200 ¾ lb. (just over 91 kilos). Walker snatched with the left hand 202¾ lb. (just over 92 kilos). Hermann's single-handed snatching ability was far in excess of that possessed by Karl Swoboda, Josef Steinbach and Josef Grafl, whose best single-handed Snatches were as follows: –

Swoboda: Right-hand Snatch , 179 ¾ lb. (81.35 kilos).

Left-hand Snatch, 168 ¼ lb. (slightly more than 76 kilos).

Steinbach: Right-hand Snatch, 189 lb. (85.7 kilos).

Left-hand Snatch, 176 ½ lb. (80 kilos).

Grafl: Right-hand Snatch, 194 ¾ lb. (88.4 kilos).

Left-hand Snatch, 180 ¾ lb. (82 kilos).

Whilst discussing Hermann's ability at single-handed Snatching, mention should be made of one of Görner's pet challenge stunts. This was a right-hand straight or stiff arm Snatch of 169¾ lb. (77 kilos) performed on a barbell with a shaft of 2 3/8 in. in diameter. Due to Hermann's tremendous gripping power, this feat was rendered impossible to others, whilst to him it was quite a simple affair.

EDGAR MÜLLER

Single-handed Jerks

On 9th November, 1919, in Leipzig, Hermann lifted 264 ½ lb. (120 kilos) in a Right-hand Clean and Jerk with Barbell. This Lift should be compared with that of the famous Russian, Georg Lurich, who, lifting in Prague, put up 266 ¾ lb. (121 kilos), but in Lurich's Lift the Bar was taken to the shoulders with two hands, whereas in Hermann's case it was lifted with the right hand only. The present World Amateur Heavy Weight Record is held by Brunstedt of Sweden, who lifted 259 lb. on 2nd December, 1948. On 21st September, 1913, in Kassel, Hermann actually cleaned and jerked with the right hand a Barbell weighing no less than 286 ½ lb. (130 kilos). The bar was jerked to arms length, but owing to faulty balance it was not 'fixed'.

For comparison with other famous Lifters, may be mentioned the best recorded Lift of Arthur Saxon, 229 ¼ lb. (104 kilos); that of Karl Swoboda of Austria with 231 ¼ lb. (105 kilos), but in this case he lifted with two hands to the shoulder; Josef Steinbach, also of Austria, lifted 233¾ lb. (106 kilos) whilst Karl Mörke lifted 248 lb. (112½ kilos), but, once again, using two hands to the shoulder.

On the Left-hand Clean and Jerk, Hermann has lifted 220 ½ lb. (100 kilos) against the best known Lift of Charles Rigoulot, the famous French Lifter, of 198½ lb. (90 kilos). Karl Swoboda, Josef Steinbach, Josef Grafl, also lifted the same weight, namely 198½ lb. It should be noted, however, that, in the case of Swoboda and Grafl, they each used two hands in taking the barbell to the shoulder, only Steinbach lifting it 'clean'.

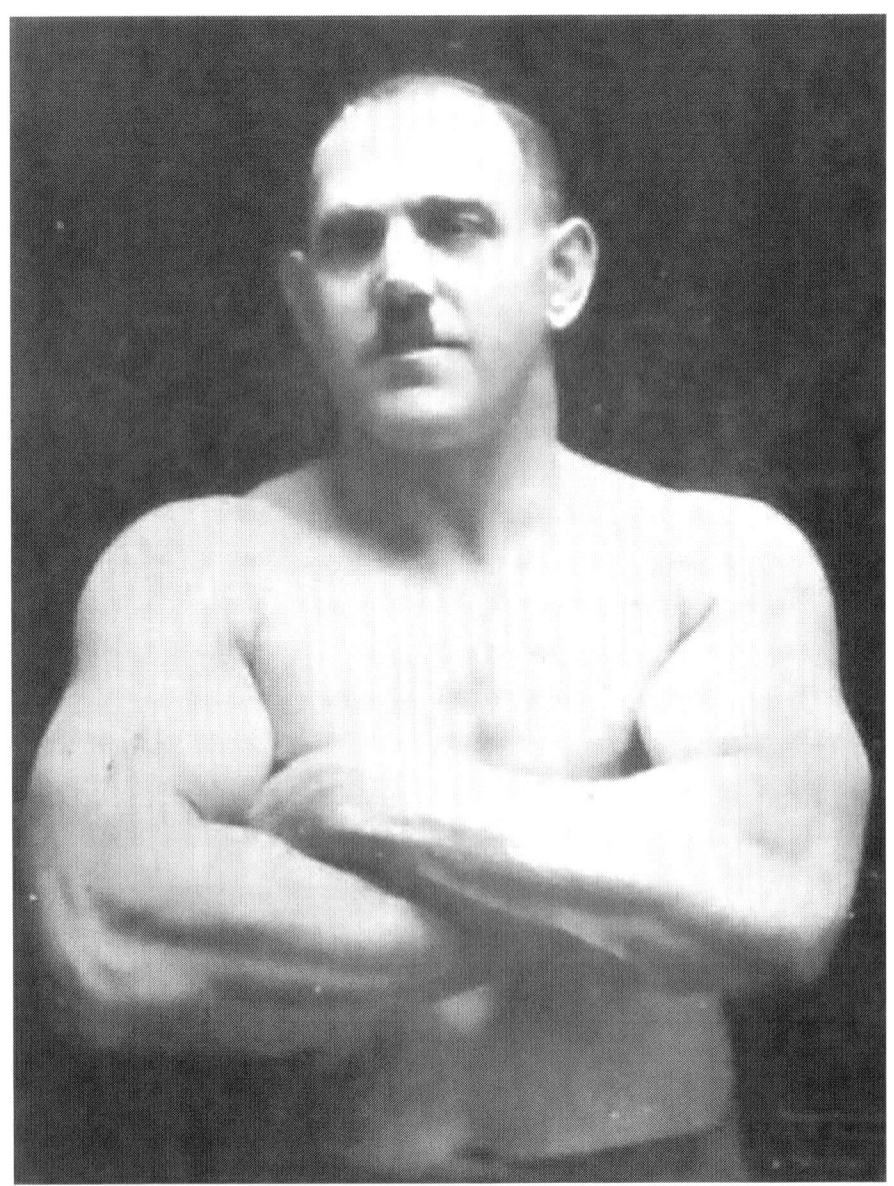

Hermann Görner in the well known "folded arms" pose. Note tremendous forearm development.

Edgar Müller

Double-Handed Jerks and 'Anyhow' Lifts

At Dresden on 25th July, 1920, Görner lifted the enormous weight of 430 lb. (a little more than 195 kilos) overhead in the Two Hands 'Anyhow' style, performing the feats with four kettleweights in the following manner. He first of all swung with the right hand two kettleweights, one weighing 110¼ lb. and the other 99¼ lb. Still holding the bells overhead, he then bent down and picked up with the left hand a third kettleweight weighing 110¼ lb. (50 kilos), which he then swung to arms length and transferred to the thumb of the right hand. Then, still holding the three kettleweights overhead in his right hand, he lowered his body carefully and with the left hand picked up the fourth kettleweight, which he slowly swung to arms length. The combined weight then held overhead for the referee's court was, as has been stated, no less than 430 English lb. or more than 195 kilos. This was a truly stupendous feat of strength. The French giant, Apollon, was stated to have swung 4 kettleweights, grasped together, with his right arm, but these weights totalled only 176 lb. or exactly 80 kilos, whereas Hermann swung with his right hand, at the commencement of the feat, two kettleweights totalling 209½ lb. (95 kilos)! Hermann then followed this colossal right-arm swing by swinging to arms length the two additional bells each weighting 50 kilos or 110¼ English lb., as has been described. For comparison with this amazing feat of Hermann's may be mentioned the great Arthur Saxon's lift of 445 ¼ lb. (202 kilos), which was performed, however, with a Barbell and a single Kettlebell. The Barbell weighed 335 lb. and the Kettlebell 110¼ lb., the lift being performed in Leipzig on 3rd November, 1905. So far as is known, that is the only recorded 'Anyhow' Lift to exceed Hermann's Lift with four Kettlebells. However, even famous Arthur Saxon, when lifting Kettleweights in the 'Anyhow' style could not exceed 300 lbs. which consisted of two Kettle-weights of 150 lb. each. No man in the world has ever lifted more weight in the shape of Kettle-weights in the 'Anyhow' style than Hermann Görner.

In the Two Hands Jerk with Barbell, Hermann has performed some stupendous Lifts, among the best of these being the following: –

411 lb. lifted at Oldham, England, on 23rd January, 1928, when he jerked from behind the neck a Barbell with a man sitting on each end, the total weight being as stated, 411 lbs. The Bar was jerked to arms length and still holding it overhead, Hermann revolved his body three times in succession, afterwards lowering the weight to the floor.

On 11th July, 1920, in Dresden, Hermann lifted in the Two Hands Clean and Jerk with Barbell 390 ¼ English lb. (177 kilos). It should be stressed that both in the 'Clean' and 'Jerk' very little splitting or squatting was resorted to. In all Lifts of this type, Hermann merely gave a very slight dip, when receiving weight in the shoulders and again when jerking overhead.

For comparison with Hermann's Lift, the best recorded Two Hands Clean and Jerk of other famous Strong Men are as follows: –

Arthur Saxon – 311 lb. This weight was jerked twice, once from the chest and once from behind the neck.

The great Ronald Walker of Wakefield, former British Heavy Weight Amateur Champion, lifted 363 ¾ lb. (165 kilos) in this style. (Unofficially 374 lb.)

The world-famous Egyptian amateur, El Saied Nosseir, lifted 368 ¼ lb.

Arnold Luhaäär of Estonia lifted 369 ¼ lb/ (167 ½ kilos).

Steve Stanko of U.S.A. lifted officially 382 lb.

Jakof Kutsenko of the U.S.S.R. in 1947 lifted 383 ½ lb.

The world professional record is held by Charles Rigoulot of France who, lifting on a specially-constructed Barbell, Cleaned and Jerked the stupendous poundage of 402 ½ lb. (182.5 kilos). This feat was performed on 1st February, 1929, in Paris. It is said that Rigoulot had nine successive failures before he was successful in lifting the weight on his tenth attempt.

It is interesting to note that so far back as 1920 Hermann Görner had lifted the colossal poundage of 390¼ lb., which compares with the World Amateur Heavy Weight Record, performed 28 years later, when the American John Davis, lifting in London at the 1948 Olympic Games, accomplished a Two Hands Clean and Jerk of 391¼ lb. (Increased to 393¼ lb. by Davis himself in October, 1950, lifting in Germany after the 1950 World's Championships in Paris.) The former German Amateur Heavyweight Champion, Josef Manager, jerked from the shoulders a barbell of 401½ lb. (182 kilos) in New York City on 25th June, 1938, on the occasion of the German Weightlifting Teams' visit to America.

The following feats will show the tremendous power possessed by Görner in Double-handed Overhead Lifting. On 7th February, 1914, he lifted in a Two Hands Clean and Jerk 335 lb. (152 kilos) consisting of a Kettleweight weighing 169¾ lb. in the right hand and a Dumbbell weighing 165 ¼ lb. in the left hand.

Hermann also made the following Lift with his heels together throughout and at no time during the Lift did his feet move from the original position of 'attention'. On 5th May, 1932, at Leipzig he cleaned and jerked a Barbell weighing 341¾ lb. (155 kilos). The bar was actually cleaned to the height of the mouth, lowered to his shoulders and without moving his feet from the original 'heels together' position the weight jerked overhead mostly by sheer arm and shoulder strength. He has also cleaned a Barbell weighing 330¾ lb. (150 kilos) to the shoulders and jerked overhead, then lowered the Bar to the 'hang' position, cleaned it again and jerked a second time overhead. Throughout this feat his feet remained together.

On 1st February, 1927, lifting in Leipzig on his Barbell with a shaft 2 3/8 in. in diameter, he lifted in the two hands Clean and Jerk 330¾ lb. During the whole lift his feet remained stationary, a very vivid demonstration of his enormous gripping power.

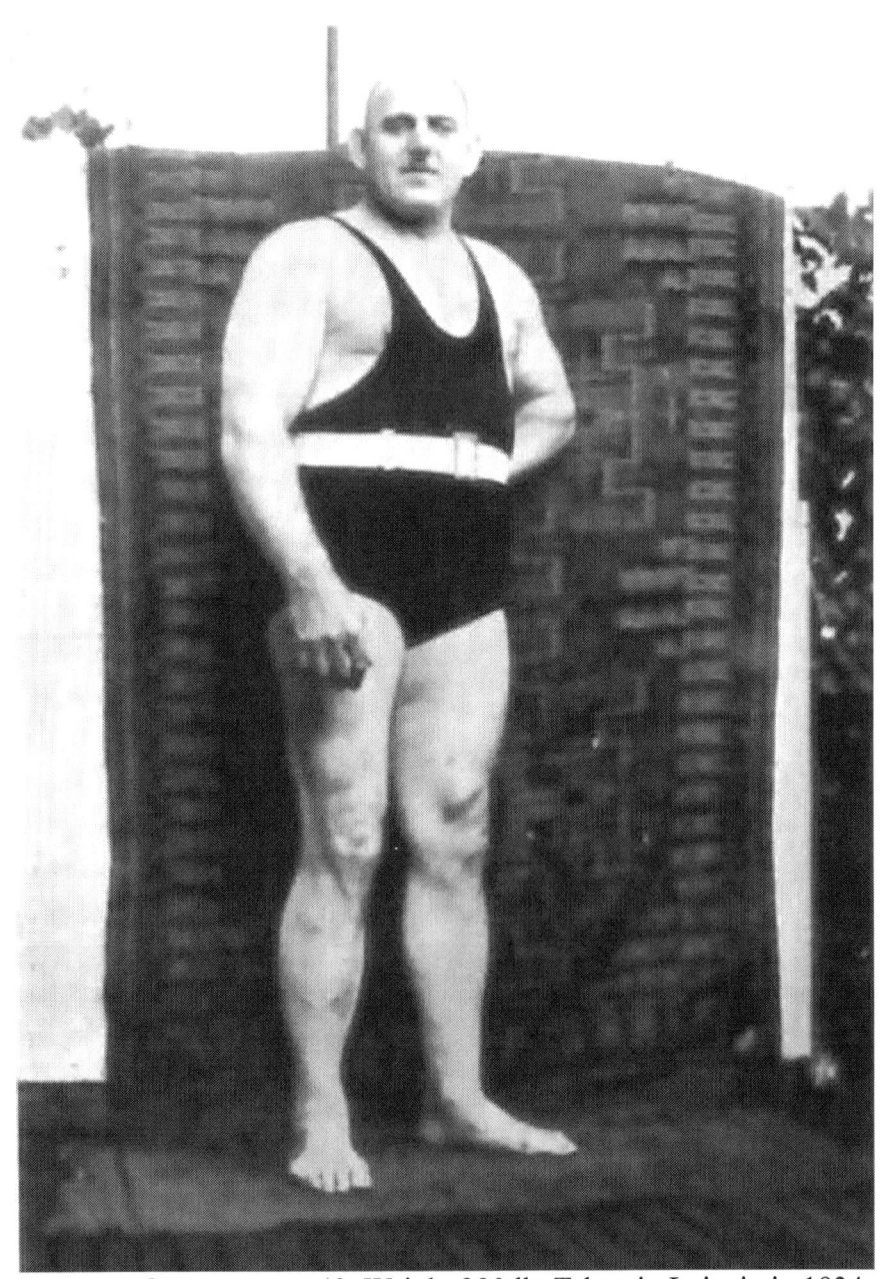

Hermann Görner at age 43. Weight 290 lb. Taken in Leipzig in 1934 by Elsie Görner.

EDGAR MÜLLER

Double-handed Snatches

Lifting at Kalk Bay, South Africa, on 4th September, 1926, Hermann snatched with two hands 297 ½ lb. This Lift of Hermann's may be compared with the late Ronald Walker's Lift of the same poundage, namely 297½ lb., although Walker is said to have unofficially snatched the tremendous weight of 320 lb. (145 kilos). The great American champion, Steve Stanko, lifted 310 lb. (140.5 kilos) when winning the Heavyweight Championship in 1941. Louis Abele, also of America, is reported to have snatched 310 lb. John Davis of U.S.A., the present World's Heavy Weight Amateur Champion holds the World's Heavyweight Record with a Lift of 327¾ lb., performed in New York on 27th January, 1950. The World's Professional Record of 315¼ lb. was established by Charles Rigoulot in 1930. In snatching, Hermann relied almost entirely on his colossal arm and shoulder strength – if he had trained to use his legs in modern style, there is no knowing what heights he might have attained. A Lift of 330 lb. would appear to have been easily possible.

A Lift which never failed to impress his audience was his performance of the Two Hands Snatch with crossed arms. When lifting in this style, Hermann gripped the Bar in the centre with his hands touching, the left arm overlapping the right. In Leipzig on 5th December, 1919, lifting in this fashion, he snatched a Barbell weighing 231½ lb. – an amazing feat of strength. He has also snatched 248 lb. whilst his feet remained in the "heels together" position throughout. This is a real 'power plus' feat!

To demonstrate his tremendous finger and gripping strength, it may be mentioned that Hermann snatched with two hands a Barbell weighing 165 ¼ lb. accomplished by merely grasping the discs at each end of the Bar. This feat was accomplished at the first attempt and was performed in Leipzig on 20th October, 1931.

Single and Double-handed Swings

In a feat of swinging weights overhead with one or two arms, Hermann was in a class by himself. The most outstanding of his many feats performed with kettleweights included the following: –

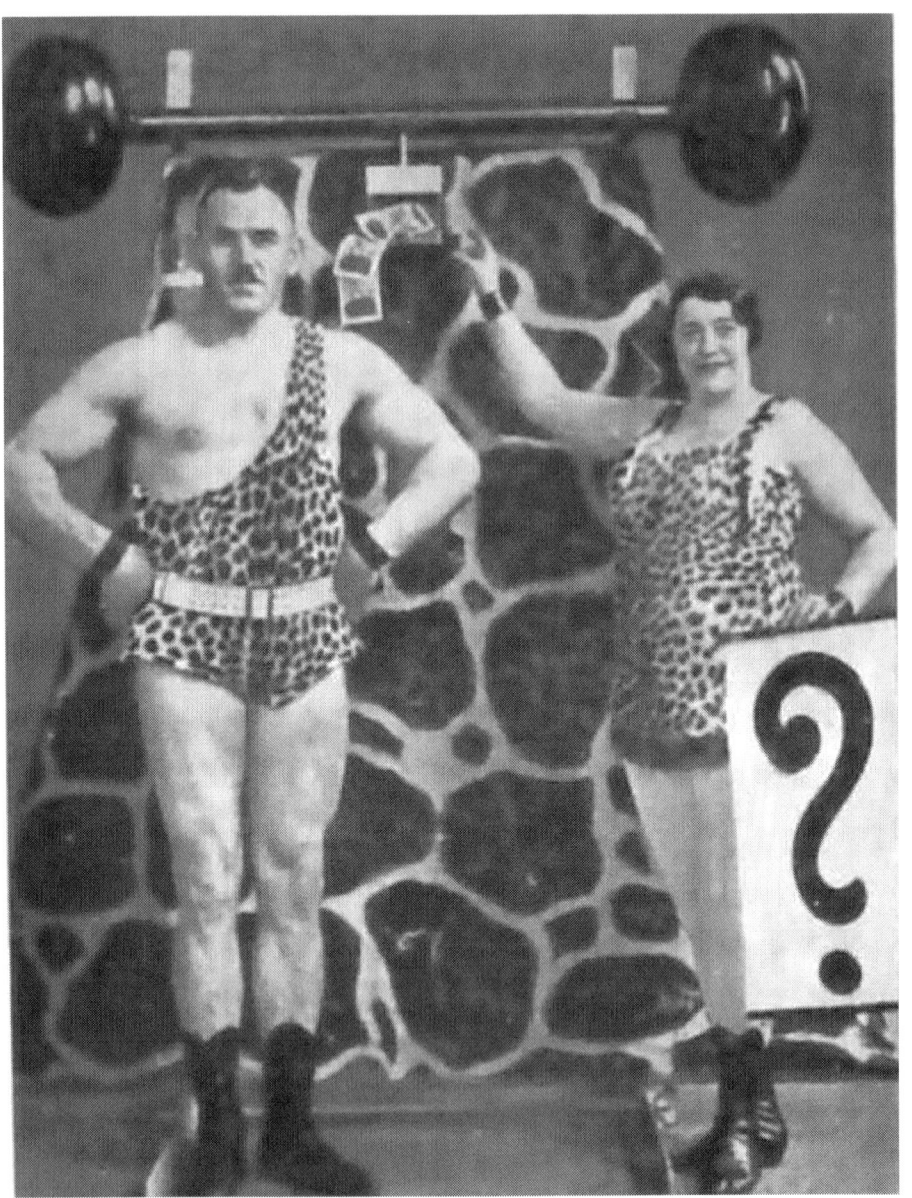

Hermann and Elsie Görner in stage costume with the famous "Challenge" barbell of 330 3/4 lb. in the background.

EDGAR MÜLLER

Right-hand Swing with two kettleweights – total weight, 187½ lb. Performed with straight arm on 5th April, 1931, in Leipzig.

Right-hand Swing with kettleweight weighing 110¼ lb. (50 kilos), swung no less than 48 times in succession. Performed on 14th July, 1912, in Leipzig.

Right-hand Swing with kettleweight weighing 132 ¼ lb., using only the forefinger of his right hand. Performed on 8th May, 1934, in Leipzig.

Right-hand Swing with kettlebell of 110 ¼ lb. (50 kilos,) using only the little finger, also performed on 8th May, 1934.

Right-hand Swing with two kettleweights (each 110¼ lb.), total weight 220½ lb. (100 kilos). Performed on 21st March, 1920, at Leipzig. (Unofficially.)

Left-hand Swing with two kettleweights – total weight 193 lb. (87½ kilos). Performed on 21st September, 1919, at Leipzig.

Right-hand Swing with two kettleweights 211¾ lb. (96 kilos). Officially performed at Leipzig on 12th October, 1919. Lifting in the same fashion Arthur Saxon performed a lift of 188½ lb. (85½ kilos) at his best.

Right-hand Swing with *three* kettleweights of equal size and shape totalling 166½ lb. (75½ kilos). Performed 5th August, 1934, at Leipzig. Arthur Saxon who possessed a larger size hand than Görner, lifted in this style three kettleweights weighing 165¼ lb. (75 kilos).

Right-hand Swing with dumb-bell weighing 150 lb. (68 kilos) *whilst sitting on a chair,* remaining seated throughout and without moving the feet. Performed at Leipzig on 4th April, 1933.

Two-hands Swing with *four* kettleweights – two in each hand – weighing 221¾ lb. (100.5 kilos) without moving the feet. The kettleweights were swung from between Görner's legs to arms length overhead. At Leipzig on 5th August, 1934.

Two-hands Repetition Swing with two kettleweights totalling 220½ lb. (100 kilos). Swung four times in succession! Performed 20th April, 1924.

Two Dumb-bells Swing. Whilst sitting on a chair Görner swung two dumb-bells weighing 200½ lb. (91 kilos) to arms length by sheer arm and shoulder strength – without raising his body from the seat or moving his feet. This amazing feat was performed on 7th March, 1933, in Leipzig.

In double-handed swinging, the following are among the outstanding feats performed by Hermann Görner in this style of lifting:–

On 26th March, 1931, lifting again in Leipzig, he swung with two kettleweights a total of 254¾ lb. This colossal feat was achieved at the first attempt and kettleweights lifted were the heaviest ones available in the Club. On this occasion, Hermann was in outstanding form and it is a matter of regret that no heavier weights were available for him to have further increased his record on this particular Lift. For comparison with this feat, the Lift of Arthur Saxon of 220½ lb., consisting of two 50-kilo kettleweights, should be mentioned. Saxon's feat was also performed in Leipzig.

Lifting with dumb-bells, Hermann has established a record of 233¾ lb. The British Heavyweight Amateur Record of this Lift stands at 225 lb., lifted by Ronald Walker of Wakefield.

Although the following feats are not swings in the accepted sense of the word, they are included because the action resembles the swing in part. These feats were all performed with kettleweights of 50 kilos or 110¼ lb. each.

Two kettleweights swung from the ground, thrown in the air and allowed to spin before being caught again by the handles, total weight 220 ½ lb.

Kettleweight of 50 kilos thrown and spun with the right hand, the bell turning *three* times on its own axis before being caught with the right hand. This feat was also performed with the left hand.

Kettleweight of 77½ kilos (171 lb.) thrown and spun and caught with the right hand. As far as is known this is believed to be the heaviest kettlebell ever juggled by any strong man in the world!

Kettleweight of 110¼ lb. (50 kilos) held in the right hand and without moving the feet thrown in shot-putting style a distance of 12 ft. 1 2/3 in.

All the above feats were performed in the months of July and August, 1934, in Leipzig.

Feats of Arm and Shoulder Strength

The following list of feats will reveal the terrific arm and shoulder strength possessed by Hermann. He is without a doubt one of the strongest armed men of all time, as a careful reading of the following feats performed by him at various times during his career will reveal.

Two-hands Hold Out with barbell

Performed on 24th March, 1933, with a barbell weighing no less than 121 ¼ lb. Lifted with straight arms from "hang" in front of body to "hold out" position and then continued to arms length overhead.

Two-hands Slow Curl sitting on floor

This feat was performed with a barbell of 209¼ lb. (95 kilos). This Lift was performed in the following manner. Hermann sat on the floor with the barbell at right angles to his thighs. From this position the weight was curled correctly to the shoulders and then pressed overhead with under-grip, with the palms of the hands facing towards the body. This feat was performed in Leipzig on 24th November, 1936.

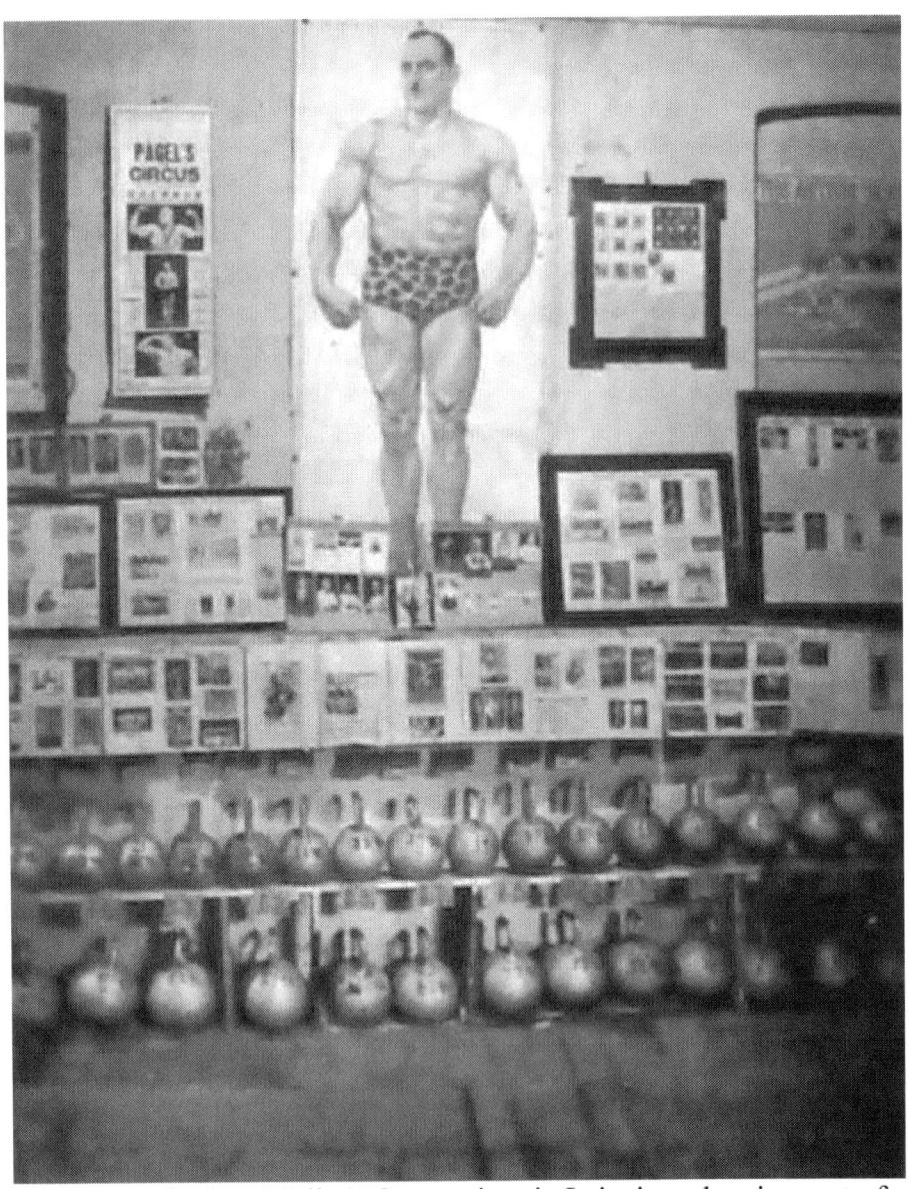

A corner of Edgar Müller's Gymnasium in Leipzig – showing part of his collection of kettleweights and photographic collection, including posters of Hermann Görner's Circus act.

EDGAR MÜLLER

Two-hands Press with two kettleweights whilst seated

In this feat Hermann sat on a chair before a table on which stood two kettleweights weighing 50 kilos (110¼ lb.) or a total of 220½ lb. The kettleweights were encircled by his hands, the thumb being placed around the kettleweight handle with the backs of the hands uppermost, the palm of the hand being in contact with the bell. From this position the arms were rotated in a half-circle, so that now the backs of his hands were touching the table top, each kettleweight being balanced in Hermann's palms. From here the bells were pulled into the shoulders and slowly pressed overhead in military style; an amazing feat of pure arm strength. Performed on 10th July, 1932, in Leipzig.

Right-hand Curl with barbell of 330 ¾ lb.

This stupendous feat was performed in the following manner. The barbell loaded to 330¾ lb. (150 kilos) was supported by two chairs. The bar being then 25½ in. from the ground. Hermann stood parallel to the bar, gripped it in the centre with his right hand and encircled his right wrist with his left hand, then with one enormous effort he 'curled' the bar into his right shoulder, standing erect at the finish of the lift. It must be stressed that this was not in any way a fast single-handed pull in, as the reader might well suppose.

Two-hands Curl with barbell

On 4th November, 1932, in Leipzig, Hermann curled with two hands a barbell weighing 242½ lb. (110 kilos). The bar was curled from the 'hang' without any body swing, using sheer arm power, but with a slight back bend.

Other feats of curling performed by Hermann are Two Hands Slow Curl with kettleweights, performed in correct English style with 220 ½ lb., consisting of 110¼ kettlebell in each hand. He has also performed a correct Two Hands Slow Curl with barbell with the same weight, namely 220½ lb. This latter lift, as far as is known, is the highest poundage ever lifted correctly in the Two Hands Slow Curl. It was performed in Leipzig on 1st September, 1932. A point that should be borne in mind by the reader is the fact that Hermann sustained a serious wound in the left forearm during the first World War, which, of course, makes his feats of arms strength all the more meritorious.

Two-hands Hold Out from below

110¼ lb. (50 kilos). Held out correctly for three seconds. Performed 14th August, 1932, in Leipzig.

Other curling feats include the following : –

A barbell of 226 lb. curled from off a table upon which was placed the barbell. Blocks 2 in. high were placed under the bar to permit hands to grasp the shaft. Elbows were rested on the table throughout the feat and the bar was curled to the shoulders, whilst Görner was seated in the chair. This movement was known in Leipzig as the 'Görner' curl. Hermann has also curled in the 'Görner' style a barbell weighing 168 lb. ten times in succession. He has also performed a Right-hand 'Görner' Curl of 121¼ lb. and 110¼ lb. with the left hand.

Rectangular Fix with barbell

Performed in Leipzig with a barbell weighing 154 ¼ lb. lifted in correct style from the 'hang' on 11th September, 1932. He has also Rectangular Fixed 160 lb., taking the barbell from off a low table.

Upright Rowing with barbell

A barbell of 286½ lb. (130 kilos) pulled up slowly from the 'hang' in military position (hands shoulder width apart) without body sway and elbows held at ear level for the count. Performed 19th October, 1931, at Leipzig.

Bend Over – or "Good Morning" Exercise

Holding a barbell of 335.8 lb. (152.35 kilos) across his shoulders – after jerking it from behind neck – Hermann did a Bendover of "Good Morning" exercise, in correct style with this

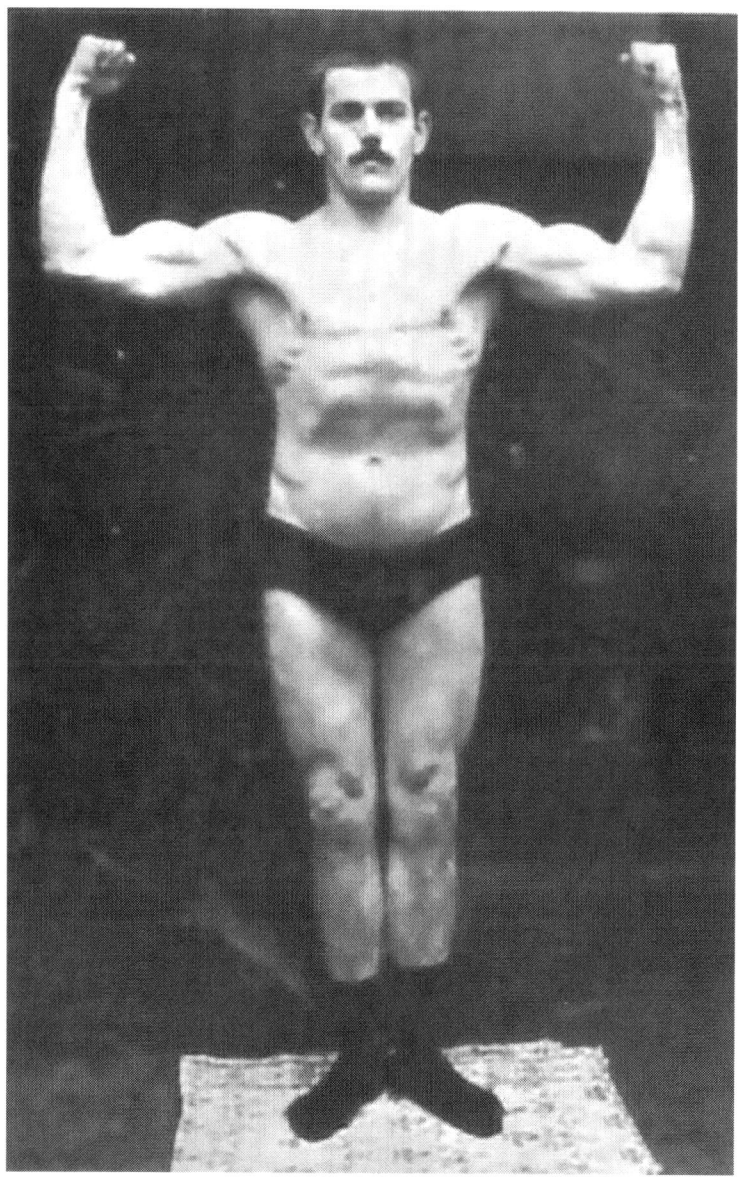

Hermann at age 17. He had already trained with weights for seven years when this was taken.

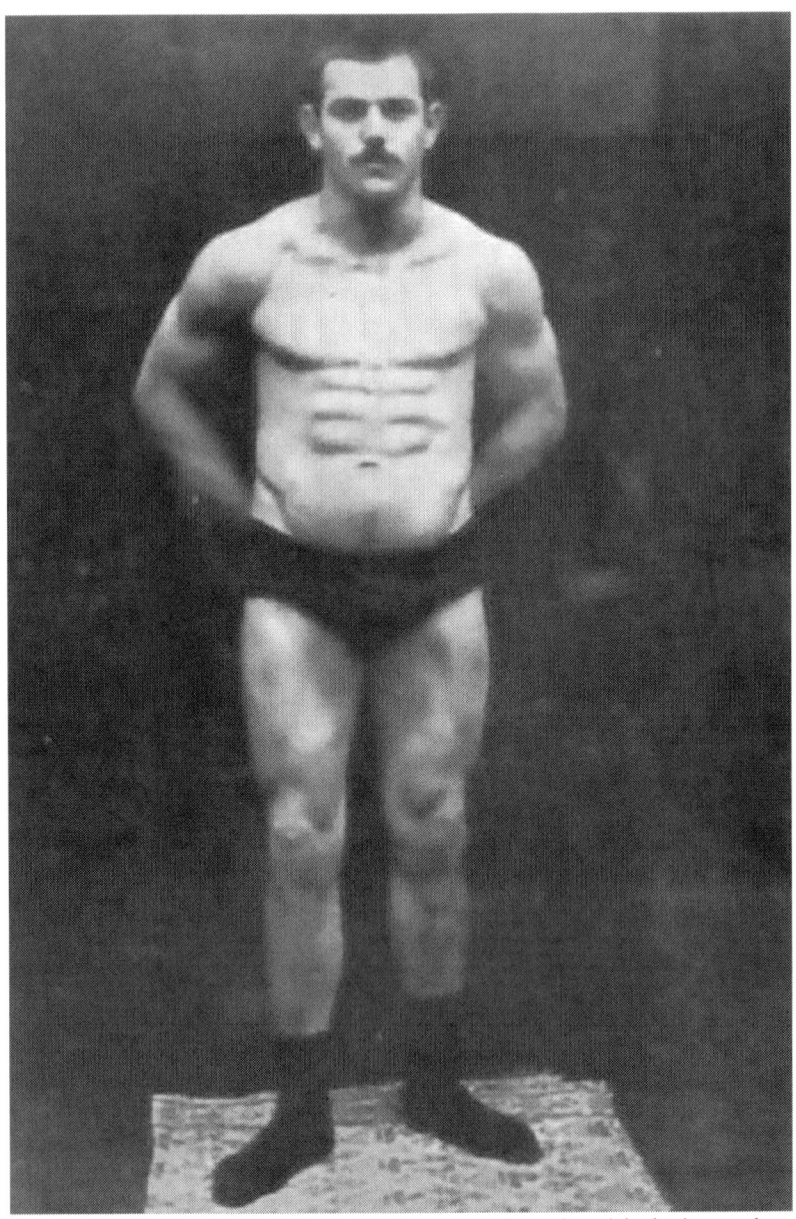

Another pose of Görner at 17 years, showing his balanced development and excellent abdominals.

tremendous weight. This was performed on 14th August, 1932, and is probably the record in this lift.

Double Handed Presses and Pushes

In perfect style Hermann often pressed 253½ lb. (115 kilos) in a Two Hands Military Press, but he did not practise this lift.

With kettleweights he has pressed 242½ lb. (110 kilos) in the Two Hands Military Press style. Using a thumbles grip, Görner did a Two Hands Push with Barbell of 286½ lb. (130 kilos) at the first attempt. It in no way represented his maximum and was performed in Leipzig on 6th June, 1933.

Supine Lifts

Hermann has accomplished the following lifts whilst lying on his back or in what is now known as the 'supine' position.

Two-hands Supine Press with barbell 330¾ lb. (150 kilos) performed in Leipzig on 26th June, 1932.

Supine Press with two barbells. A combined weight of 308½ lb. The bells pressed simultaneously. Performed 24th October, 1933, at Leipzig. This was a Lift very seldom practised by Hermann. The poundages given are well below what he could have lifted had he been sufficiently interested to train seriously for a short while on this Lift.

Lifts to Shoulders – Single and Double-handed

It is the contention of many authorities that the hallmark of a Strong Man is the amount of weight he can : –

   (a) lift off the ground, and
   (b) lift to his shoulders.

The reason being that in the performance of both these feats application of science or skill is largely eliminated – the amount that can be lifted being governed almost solely by the strength possessed by the individual. A close examination of the following feats performed during his career by Hermann Görner will reveal very vividly the enormous bodily strength and all-round power he possessed, as in all the feats listed sheer brute strength is the predominating factor in their execution.

Two-hands Barbell Lift to Shoulder

A barbell of 442¼ lb. (over 200 kilos) lifted to the shoulders in two movements – in other words, 'continentalled' to the shoulders. This was performed without squatting or splitting on 10th January, 1933, in Leipzig, and surpassed Hermann's previous record of 441 lb., which he perfoormed at Breslau on 27th July, 1913. As far as it is known, this is the heaviest weight ever to be lifted to the shoulders unassisted, although it is now some 17 years since Hermann performed this amazing feat. History has it that the giant Viennese, Karl Swoboda, lifted overhead with two hands a barbell weighing 440 lb., which, it is said, took four men to lift to his shoulders. The highest recorded feat of lifting to the shoulders unassisted appears to be Rigoulot's feat of 402¼ lb., performed on his specially-constructed barbell, although it has been reported that Charles Rigoulot performed unofficially a Two-hands Clean to the shoulders with 422 lb. (191.4 kilos), but more exact information regarding this Lift would appear to be unobtainable. John Davis of U.S.A. is said to have lifted clean to the shoulders 405 lb. (183.7 kilos). Harold Cleghorn of Auckland, New Zealand, Continental Jerked 408 lb. (185 kilos), when lifting in the Australian/ New Zealand Championship in 1942. 409¼ lb. was lifted in the two-hands Continental Jerk by Swoboda in Vienna on 4th November, 1911. It is worthy of note that, in executing his lift, Swoboda took no less than five movements to get his barbell to the shoulders before jerking it overhead.

EDGAR MÜLLER

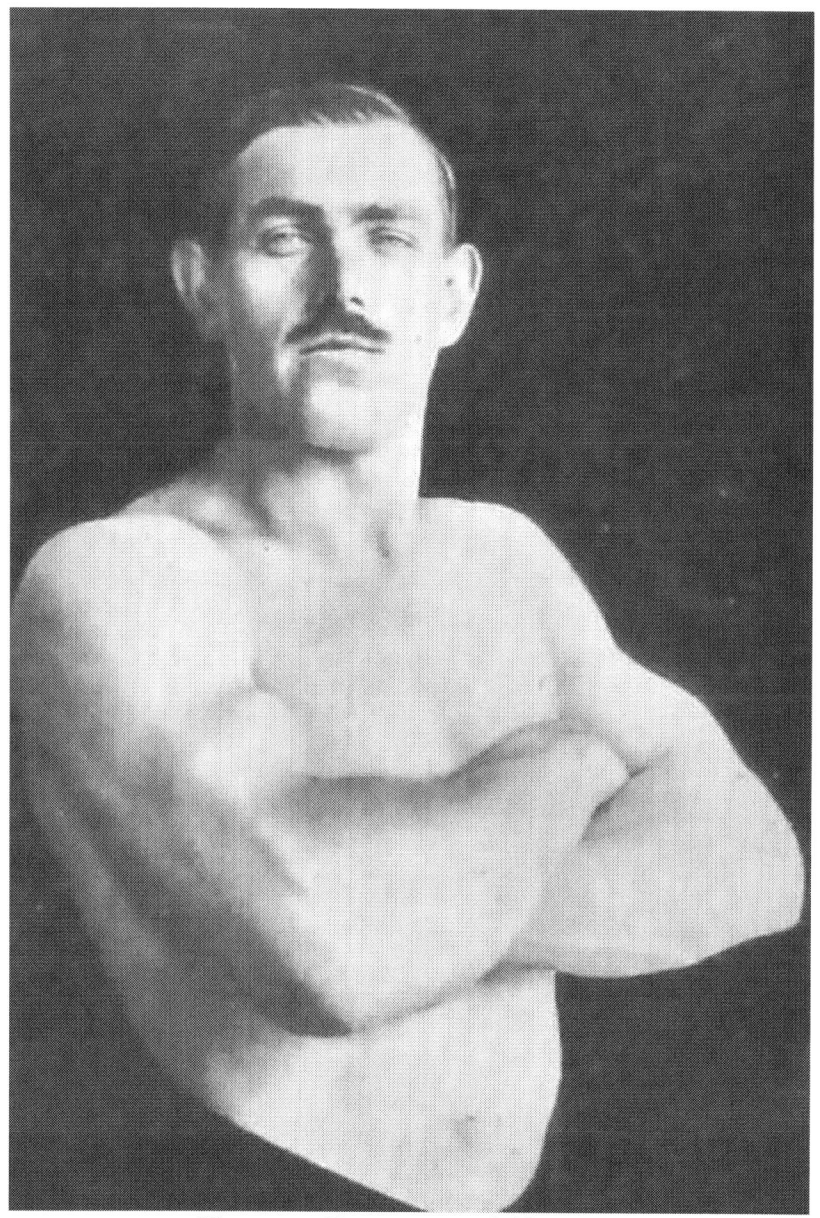

Hermann Görner – aged 18 years.

One Arm Turn In to Shoulder with barbell

In Leipzig on 25th September, 1920, Hermann upended and turned in to the shoulder with the right hand a barbell weighing no less than 385¾ lb. (175 kilos). As far as the writer is able to trace, no other man living has lifted with one arm in this style a greater weight. Arthur Saxon, who bent-pressed a barbell weighing 371 lb. to arm's length without erecting the body, used two hands in taking this bar to the shoulders, Saxon's best one-handed lift to the shoulders being 315 lb.

Right-hand Clean to Shoulder with barbell

Lifting in Leipzig on 9th November, 1919, Hermann cleaned with the right hand a barbell weighing 297½ lb. (135 kilos).

Two-hands Clean with barbell whilst sitting on chair

In Leipzig on 7th October, 1931, Hermann lifted clean from the floor to the shoulders a barbell weighing 220½ lb., whilst he himself was seated on an ordinary kitchen chair – a pretty strong one at that! In this feat, the barbell was lifted into the shoulders using pure arm and shoulder strength only. No help being obtained from the legs or back. Hermann remained seated throughout the performance.

Dead Lifting Single and Double-handed

These lifts are truly what W.A. Pullum, the well-known English Strong Man and trainer of Strong Men, once described as 'the fundamental test of a man's bodily strength'. The reading of the following feats performed by Hermann Görner will leave one in no doubt whatever that Hermann possessed 'bodily strength' to a degree it is the fortune of few mortals to own. In connection with these stupendous feats of strength, may it be recorded that Hermann could never be persuaded to train upon dead lifts, his contention being that such feats were inclined to increase the blood pressure. He lifted always within his powers – what he might have done had he been persuaded to train on these lifts can only be left to the imagination. Would 900 lb. (or more) have been beyond the bounds of possibility!

830 lb. Two-hands Dead Lift

This amazing feat was performed in Leipzig on 18th August, 1933, the weight consisting of a 441 lb. barbell and two men. Both men stood on the bar, one either end, and balanced themselves by placing their hands on Görner's shoulders. The combined weight was then lifted by Hermann who stood erect with it and held it in the correct finishing position for several seconds.

793 ¾ lb. Two-hands Dead Lift

This is believed to be still the highest poundage lifted in the orthodox style. It was performed by Hermann in Leipzig on 29th October, 1920, using an ordinary 'Berg' barbell. It is interesting to note that the bar was lifted with an overhand 'hook' grip and not the more usual reverse grip used by most lifters when executing the double-handed dead lift. The highest officially recorded two-hands dead lift approaching this stupendous feat of Hermann's is that performed by the American Light Heavy Weight Bob Peoples (body weight 189 lb. – 13 stone, 7 lb.), who lifted 725½ lb. on 4th March, 1949, at Johnson City, Tennessee, U.S.A.

The best dead lifts performed by the famous French heavyweights, Rigoulot and Cadine, were 621¾ lb. and 617¼ lb. respectively. Other outstanding dead lifts include those made by Carl Pepke, an American amateur, who lifted 657 lb. in 1947. Walter Podolak, also of America, lifted 660 lb. unofficially and 641¾ lb. officially. John Davis of U.S.A. is reported to have lifted 705 lb. (319.8 kilos) at a body weight of 190½ lb. (86.5 kilos).

734½ lb. Right-hand Dead Lift – Blockweight

This lift was made by lifting a square block of sandstone with a handle attached. The weight was lifted between the legs using the 'hook' grip, the whole block being lifted until body was erect and both legs straightened. Performed in Dresden on 20th July, 1920.

Right-hand Dead Lift with barbell

On this lift Hermann has lifted more weight than any other man in the world. His best performances being 727½ lb. (330 kilos), which was lifted unofficially on 8th October, 1920, in Leipzig. The bar was correctly lifted from the floor to the fully erect position of the body. Officially Hermann has performed a right-hand dead lift with a barbell of 663½ lb. (301 kilos), which was lifted on 29th October, 1920, in Leipzig. No other man has come within aiming distance of Hermann's amazing record. Some of the outstanding right-hand dead lifts performed include 502 lb. lifted by Laurence Chappell in 1932. Chappell being the English Amateur 12 stone lifter. The great Charles Rigoulot lifted 450 lb. in the right-hand dead lift, performed in Paris in 1926. Ernest Cadine, the French heavyweight lifted 449¾ lb. (204 kilos) in the right-hand dead lift.

Malcolm Brenner, an American heavyweight, performed a one hand dead lift of 550 lb. in October, 1949.

617¼ lb. Two-hands Dead Lift with two barbells

In performing this feat Hermann stood between two barbells which he grasped with a 'hook' grip and lifted simultaneously. The right barbell weighed 330¾ lb. (150 kilos) whilst the left-hand barbell weighed 286½ lb. (130 kilos). Both bars were lifted from the floor to the hang and held in correct erect finishing position for three seconds. The feat being performed in Leipzig on 9th November, 1934.

595¾ lb. Four Finger Two-hands Dead Lift

This lift was made by Hermann using the first two fingers of each hand only. It was not regarded in any way as his maximum and was lifted by him purely as a demonstrating lift

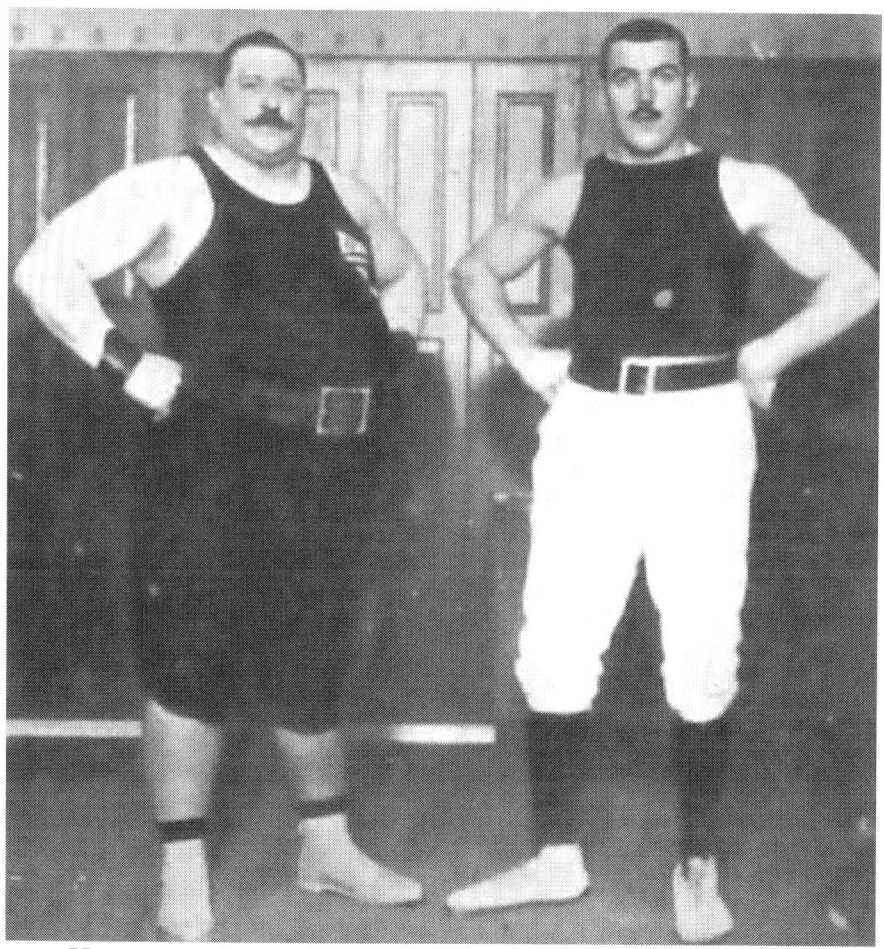

Hermann Görner with Karl Swoboda, World's Heavyweight Champion. Photograph taken in Leipzig on 21st September 1912 when Hermann was just over 21 years old. Swoboda was 30 years old and weighed 342 lb.

on 30th November, 1933, in Leipzig.

Two-hands 'Bent Arm' Dead Lift

Using a grip with the over-hand style and both arms half bent at right angles to the floor, the bar being lifted from the floor to waist high, Hermann has raised a barbell weighing 441 lb., performed 5th May, 1932, in Leipzig.

SUPPORTING FEATS, INCLUDING FEATS OF LEG AND BODILY STRENGTH

The following performances have been established by Hermann at various stages of his career and clearly demonstrate his all-round bodily strength, when applied to supporting feats and other feats performed in lifting heavy and awkward objects, carrying and supporting enormous weights in various positions.

The 'Plank' Feat

This feat which was also a favourite with Arthur Saxon in his act was performed by Görner on many occasions. It was usually included as a regular item in his nightly circus performance and on 12th October, 1927, in London, he performed this feat with a total of 4,123 lb. which weight was made up of 24 men sitting on a plank which, in turn, was supported on the soles of the feet whilst Hermann was lying on his back. In his nightly performance, Hermann allowed 16 men to sit on the plank and never at any time paid any heed to the weights of each volunteer. In this feat it was said that Arthur Saxon had supported a weight of 3,200 lb. with a total of 20 men.

The 'Human Bridge' Support

This extraordinary and dangerous feat consisted of carrying the entire weight of a motor-car holding six men, which was driven over a specially constructed bridge under which Hermann stood forming the human support at one end, the bridge resting on his shoulders as he stood erect under it. The weight of the car and passengers totalled 4,000 lb. Görner was the only man in the world to practise this outstanding supporting feat. During his tour with Pagel's in South Africa, he performed a similar feat except that here the bridge was supported by his feet whilst Hermann was lying on his back beneath the bridge. The car, in this instance, being a Mercedes Benz carrying seven passengers. This supporting feat was also once featured by the Saxon brothers in their act, but in their case two of the brothers acted as the human support of the bridge by lying beneath it on their backs and carrying the weight on their four legs. In Hermann's case, he took the entire weight alone. The only other man known to have featured a similar act solo is the German Strong Man and Wrestler, Henry Steinborn.

The 'Merry-Go-Round' Support

This feat consisted of supporting a small Merry-Go-Round on which eight persons enjoyed a ride. Hermann supported on his feet whilst lying on his back the whole contraption, which weighed in excess of 2,300 lb. This feat was performed nightly during his stay in England and during his tours of South Africa.

'Tomb of Hercules' Feat

This feat performed with a platform resting on knees and chest, whilst Hermann reclined on a box holding up the platform on which twelve persons were standing, was performed nightly in 1927, when he was in England, at the conclusion of a stage act in which as the opening piece six dancing girls performed a ballet dance on the platform supported by Hermann. The whole platform with this load was supported by Görner for as long as eight minutes on occasions.

Lifting a Car with Driver

This feat was performed as an impromptu feat of strength by Hermann in 1920, when grasping the front axle of a

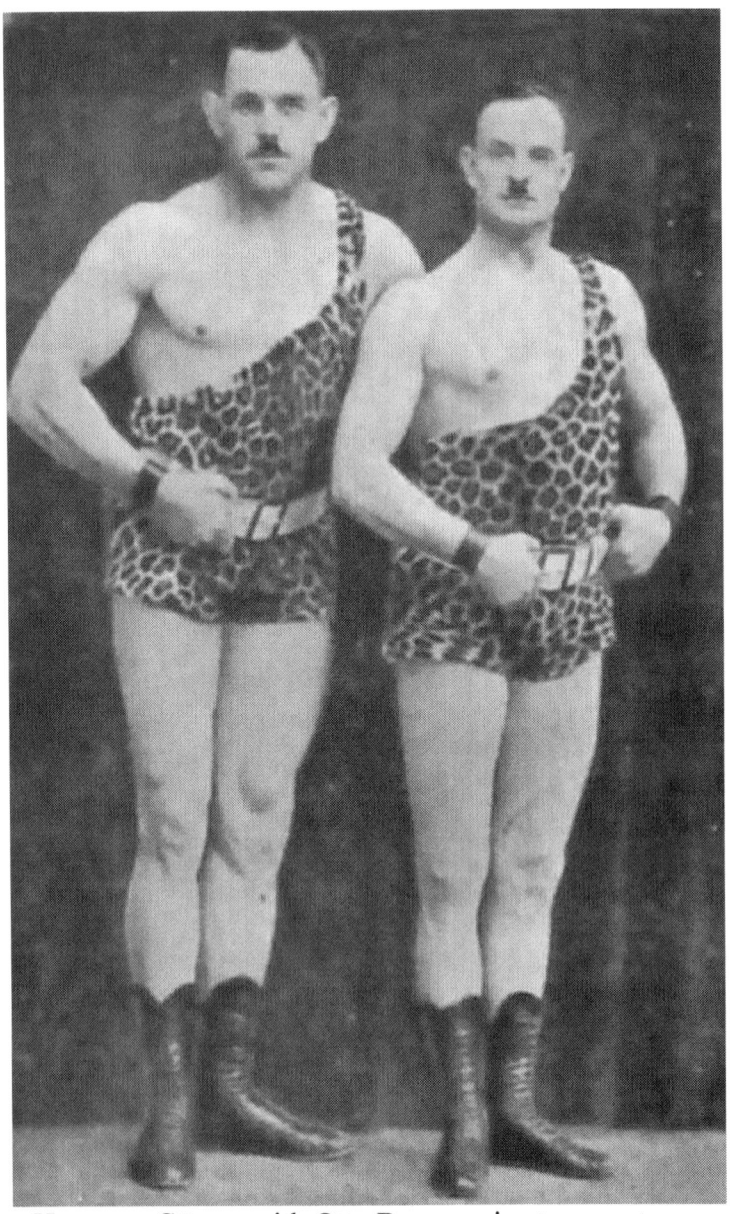

Hermann Görner with Otto Brauer – in stage costume.

car in which the driver was seated, Hermann stood erect and then walked in a semi-circle carrying the weight of the car with him, whilst the two rear wheels rested on the ground. The total weight was 3,042½ lb. and the poundage actually lifted was estimated to work out at 1,362 ½ lb. Performed 25th September, 1920.

Resisting the Efforts of Sixteen Men

This feat was performed whilst Hermann was in England in 1927 and was carried out by Hermann climbing ten steps of a ladder whilst sixteen men unsuccessfully endeavoured to pull him down by means of a rope attached to his body and held by the men "tug-o'-war" fashion.

Carrying a Grand Piano

As a result of a wager, Hermann had a grand piano weighing 1,444 lb. strapped to his back after which he successfully essayed a walk of 52½ feet. This amazing stunt was carried out in Leipzig on 3rd June, 1921. Needless to say, Herman won his wager!

Carrying 100 Bricks – Weight over 1,000 lb.

This feat was carried out by stacking 100 bricks into a special hod the whole load then being taken from the trestle and carried on his shoulders up the staircases of a piano factory in Leipzig, performed on 10th May, 1912. The total weight being 1,124 ½ lb.

Walking with over 1,000 lb. on the Shoulder

This feat was performed by carrying on the right shoulder a special bar to which was attached two barrels, on each barrel being two men. The total weight was 1,104½ lb. The bar with its load was lifted and shouldered off the ground and then Hermann walked the length of the circus arena and twirled round before replacing the whole load on the ground. This extraordinary feat was performed by Hermann at every performance during his stay with Pagel's circus in Capetown,

South Africa, in 1935.

Walking and Carrying 661 lbs.

This feat was performed every evening during his Music Hall performance in England in 1927. Hermann wore full evening dress and carried in each hand a heavy travelling trunk, the trunks opened and revealed two chorus girls inside each one. Hermann would walk on to the stage, carrying the trunks nonchalantly. After walking the length of the stage and turning round, he would put the trunks down, whereupon the lids of the trunks opened to reveal the four dancing girls he had so easily carried.

Feats of Combined Agility and Strength

Hermann picked up four kettleweights two in each hand, a total of 441 lb., and then ran with them round the training hall in Leipzig, a distance of 78 feet. This feat was performed on 5th August, 1934. On another occasion, many years previously, on 2nd June, 1912, he sprinted 100 metres (109 yds. 13 in.) in 18.4 seconds, whilst carrying in each hand a kettlebell weighing 50 kilos, or a total weight of 220½ lb. How about trying this some time!

Before closing this formidable catalogue of some of Hermann's amazing performances, the following should also be mentioned.

He has written his name on a blackboard with a kettleweight of no less than 110¼ lb. (50 kilos) dangling from his thumb!

He has performed with a full-grown man what is known as the 'Puppet Dance'. That is, the person lifted was grasped by the elbows by the lifter – both facing the same way – and then swung from side to side. Throughout the feat the 'puppet' is held off the ground. Hermann has performed this using as his puppet the person of Landlord Hans Preusser of Leipzig, who weighed no less than 336¼ lb. Hermann handled him as an ordinary Strong Man would a woman of 6 stone.

EDGAR MÜLLER

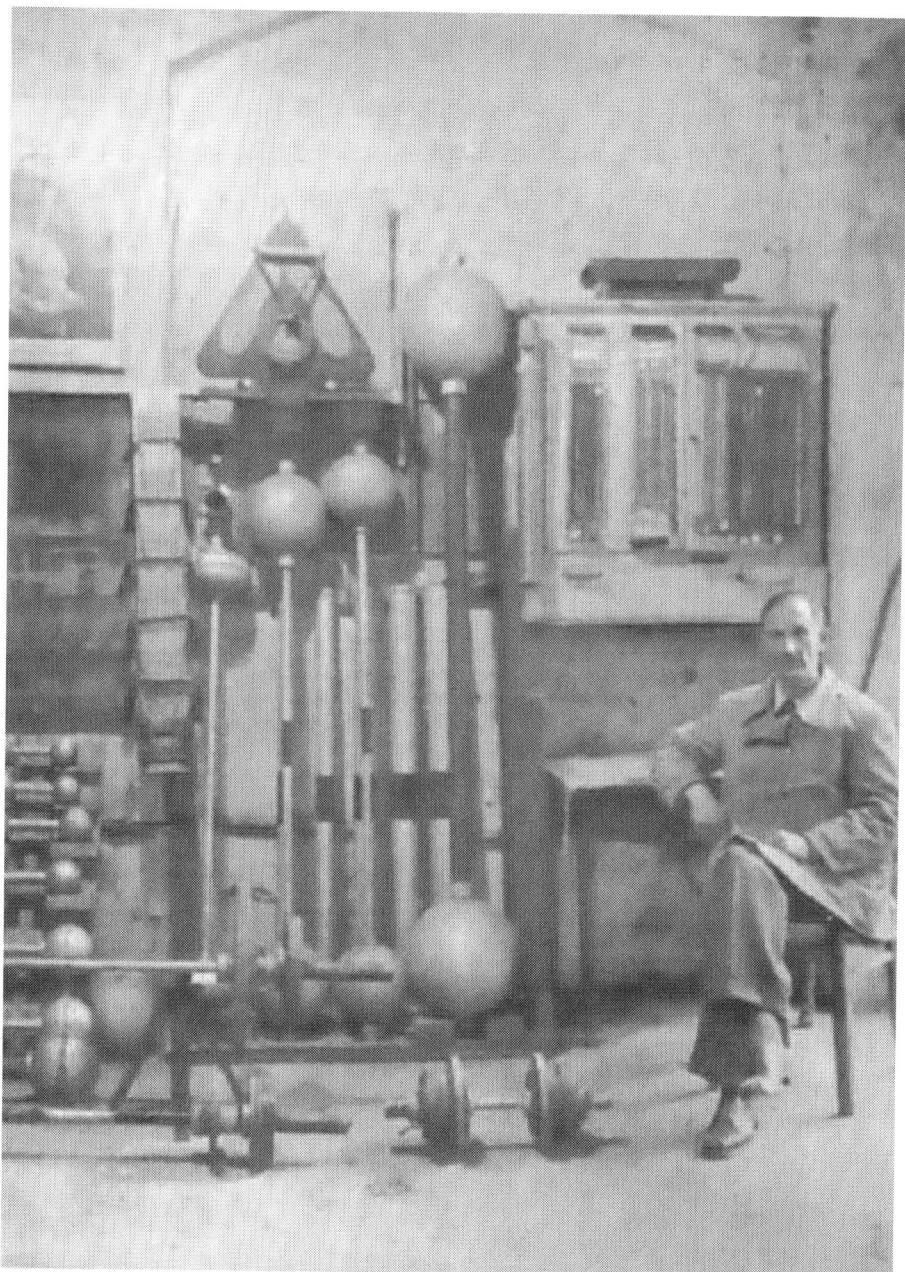

Edgar Müller, the Author of this book, in a corner of his Gymnasium in Leipzig, showing part of his collection of training equipment.

Holding a bar behind his neck on which two men were sitting, one at each end he has jerked this overhead and then a third man has performed a hand-stand on the centre of the bar. The total weight thus supported overhead by Hermann being 449¾ lb. This feat was performed on 25th January, 1920, in Leipzig.

Hermann has lifted a beer barrel of 200 litres which weighed no less than 595¾ lb. This he has lifted from the floor and placed on one end upon a table, thus winning a wager. Performed 9th July, 1910.

He has performed a Deep Knee Bend with 474¼ lb. The barbell being held in front of the body at the shoulders. This was performed in Leipzig on 11th May, 1920. Hermann was not fond of deep knee bending and hardly ever practised this lift. With his enormous bodily power it can be reasonably assumed that had he put in some time training on the Deep Knee Bend, he would have been capable of a poundage approaching 600. With all his feats performed after World War I, it must be remembered that he still had many shrapnel fragments embedded in his legs. If one examines closely the photograph on page 43, a dark spot can be seen just above his left knee. This was a piece of shrapnel which later worked through the skin and was removed by Hermann himself!

EDGAR MÜLLER

CHAPTER 6

His Training Methods

THIS chapter describes for the first time the training methods of Hermann Görner which he used so successfully in developing his enormous all-round bodily strength. It is believed that a careful study of his methods as related in this chapter will not only prove of great interest to readers but will also provide the seeker after strength (with a capital "S"!) with a method which he may use to his personal advantage – modified of course to suit the individual requirements of the serious Strength student.

As one would expect from the recital of his many different feats of strength, the training of Görner was of an all-round and varied nature and covered feats and exercises with weights in every conceivable manner. For convenience, I have decided to split up this chapter into sections each dealing with a phase of training, and in these sections I will endeavour to deal as thoroughly as possible with Hermann's methods – which, I might add, were also the methods I myself laid down in my own Gymnasium in Leipzig.

NUMBER OF TRAINING SESSIONS AND DURATION

The number of training sessions per week varied during Görner's career. Between the years 1905 to 1913 he trained usually five times per week, with two days of complete rest. These five sessions included two in the open air (during the summer months) when he trained on the Sporting Beach of the Germania Bath in Leipzig. This was a large open-air swimming pool with a beach adjoining which was supplied with a very full and varied assortment of training apparatus – barbells, dumb-bells, kettleweights, parallel bars, horizontal bars and other equipment. During this same period (1905 to 1913) there were also periods when Hermann trained daily. After the end of World War I, from 1919 to 1921, Görner trained on an average four times per week, which included one or two weekly open-air training sessions at the

Germania Bath.

During Hermann Görner's professional career – from 1921 onwards – he practised daily with the weights. After the age of 40, when not professionally engaged, he trained three times weekly – for the book, it may be recorded that his training days were usually Tuesdays and Fridays in the evening and on Sunday mornings.

Each training session averaged two hours when performed in the Club, and when training in the open air it would vary between three and four hours – sometimes even longer. It may be a matter of interest to note that when training in the open air at the Germania Bath, Hermann would sometimes conclude his training by having a swim, and at other times he would take a swim first and then carry out his training with the weights. He would not dry himself after bathing but permit his body to dry by the action of sun and air upon it. In this respect, it is interesting to record that the great George Hackenschmidt also used the same method in his training. This mixing of swimming and weightlifting may seem somewhat unusual to many readers, as I have often read that training with weights does not mix well with swimming – in Hermann's case it certainly did! Some of his swims would be short – of ten or so minutes duration – and at other times he would be in the water for an hour or more. He trained always as the mood took him – varying his programme to suit his energy and condition of the moment and never did he force himself to perform any workout when not feeling just in the mood. Incidentally, in passing, it may be mentioned that the famous Arthur Saxon also trained many times in the open air at the Germania Bath.

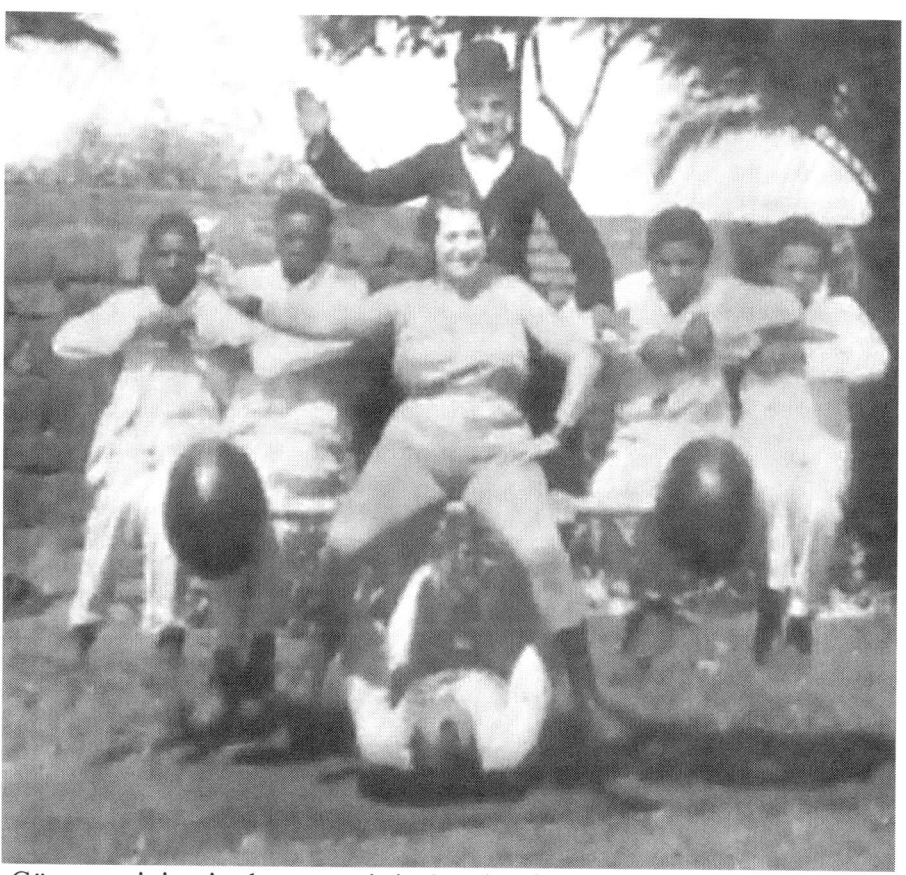

Görner training in the open air in South Africa – Elsie Görner is seated on the barbell, which weighs 330 3/4 lb.

A Typical Training Programme

In giving details of a typical training programme of Hermann Görner's, may I preface this with the comment that this is an extremely difficult thing to do, for the simple reason that he did not have or follow what might be really termed a "set" training programme – he always varied his workouts and mixed his work so much that one could truthfully say that he never worked through exactly the same programme twice. He did, of course, use a planned and progressive programme but he did not, as many do, map out a certain number of lifts with a certain poundage and then perform them a set number of times for a given period. Each training session of Hermann's contained a mixed programme of kettle-bell, dumb-bell and barbell lifting. Sometimes a workout would also include supporting feats. For instance, when Hermann trained three times per week, he might in the first training session give preference to kettlebell exercises, but he would also include barbell and dumb-bell lifts too. The second session might see the emphasis placed on dumb-bell training with not so much on kettlebell and barbell work, and the third workout would have the emphasis placed on barbell work with just a little kettlebell and dumb-bell work included in the session. During his open-air training periods at the Germania Bath, his workouts would also include putting the shot, weight-throwing, jumping and swimming in addition to working out with the weights. It would be fair to say that kettleweight training played a very large part in Görner's workouts.

As I have already said, it would be quite impossible to lay down a certain set of lifts and say, "These lifts were practised by Görner with such-and-such weights, so many repetitions, for so many weeks." He simply did not train that way. His inventive mind was always scheming out new and different ways of lifting all kinds of weights – kettlebells, dumb-bells, barbells, block weights, barrels, loaded sacks, etc. It is no wonder that Hermann forgot what his personal records were at any one of the many hundreds of feats he had performed with weights. Whenever he wished to surpass a particular feat of his, he would ask me at each training session: "Edgar, what was my best feat at such-and-such a lift?". I would refer to my Record Book and Hermann would be informed how much he had lifted on that particular occasion and on that particular lift. Usually, after this prompting, Hermann would recall the lift and when he made it – he would then proceed to better that particular feat, but he would never try his limit. He was always most "economical" with his enormous strength and, due to this, very many of his lifts were nowhere near his maximum ability – for instance, his feats of Supine Pressing, to quote just one example.

It need hardly be stressed that Görner was Leipzig's greatest attraction in "Iron Game" circles and very many officials, lifters and strength-followers from other Leipzig clubs visited our Club at nearly every training session for witessing Görner working out and for observing at first hand every movement of this living "Muscle Mountain". It is no wonder that Leipzig and other Weightlifting Clubs engaged Görner for their Exhibition Shows, knowing full well that 3000 to 4000 spectators would show up to see Görner in the flesh. As a matter of passing interest, it may be mentioned that Leipzig alone had 34 weightlifting Clubs throughout the city.

Now to try to describe an average workout of Görner's which he would do in the Leipzig Club in an evening – a workout lasting about two hours. He would usually start by working out through what in Germany we call "Die Kette" – The Chain – but this is no ordinary chain. Let me try and describe it for you. Down one side of the gymnasium is a row of kettleweights – a total of nineteen – the first one weighing 13 kilos (about 28.5 lb.) and the last one 52.5 kilos (about 115.75 lb.). The whole row of kettlebells were paired off, except the last and heaviest one, giving a gradual increase of approximately 5 to 10 lb. per pair. The final pair of kettle-weights weighing 220.5 lb. (100 kilos) together. The kettleweights were placed in a row on the floor of the gymnasium, and working "Die Kette" (or The Chain) meant that Hermann would start out by taking the first kettleweight in the right hand and swinging it to arm's length overhead, after swinging it, the weight would be lowered to the shoulder and then pressed up again overhead, relowered to the shoulder and from there to the "hang" and then curled to the shoulder, then pressed overhead again and finally lowered again and replaced on the floor. He would then repeat this with

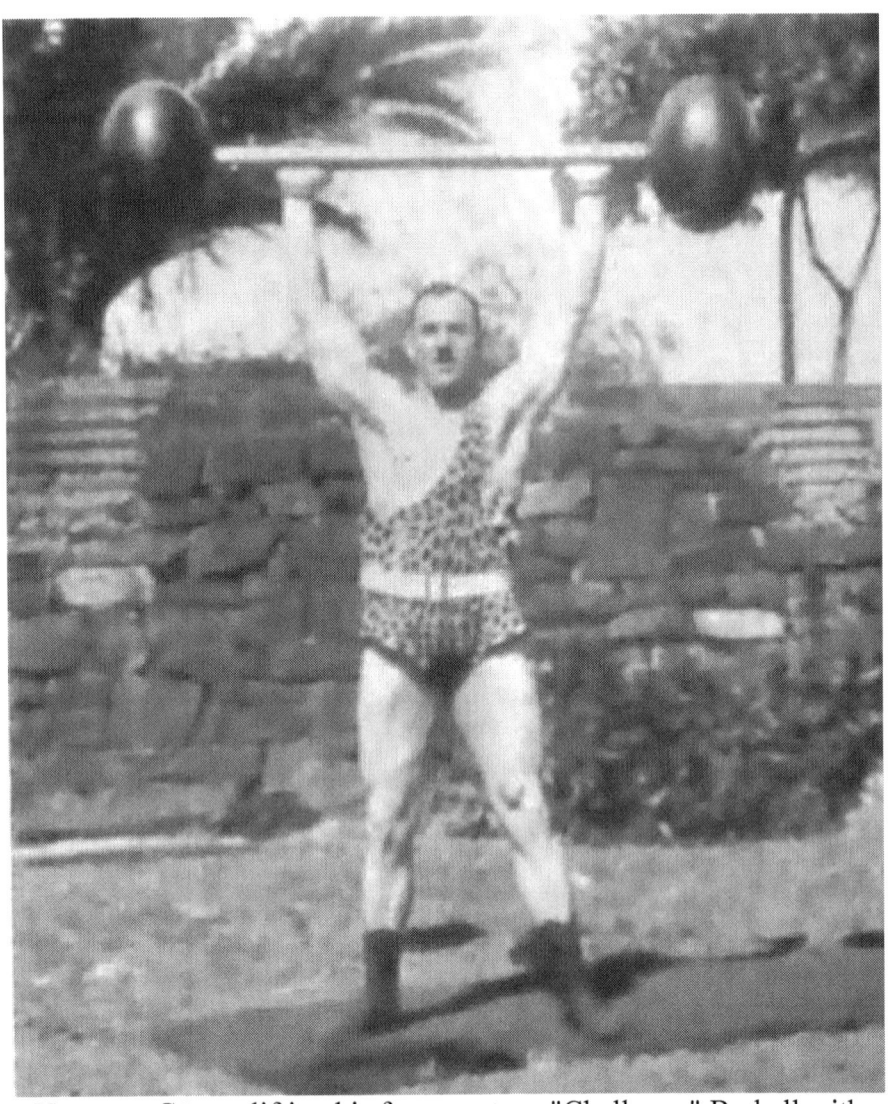

Hermann Görner lifting his famous stage "Challenge" Barbell with shaft of 2 3/8 in. diameter and weighing 330¾ lb. (150 kilos). Photograph taken in Cape Town, South Africa in 1923.

the next kettleweight, using this time the left hand. The whole length of The Chain would be worked through in this manner – in Hermann's case he would lift all the bells in this fashion with the exception that he did not curl the last and final kettleweight of 115.74 lb. – but he could curl both the 110.25 (50 kilos) kettleweights! Other members of the Club would work through The Chain as far as possible – stopping only when limited by their strength.

At other times, Hermann would work through The Chain and vary the method of working out – for instance, he might perform only Swings with each arm – he might do Swings with both arms, taking a pair of the kettleweights at the same time – he might Swing a pair of the bells singlehanded grasping them both in one hand – he might Swing the weights held on the palm of the hand – Swing them from between the legs or outside the legs – again he might work through doing the Two Hands Anyhow, sometimes Swinging each weight, sometimes Pressing each weight overhead. This working through The Chain might take up the first forty minutes of his work-out. At times, he would practise also Cleaning and Swinging on *one* leg, with either hand in turn, starting with the right leg when working with the right arm and vice versa with his left arm. Throughout the Clean or the Swing, he would be balanced entirely on one leg until the bell was replaced on the floor.

The second forty minutes might then be taken up by working out in similar fashion with dumb-bells, and the final forty minutes would be occupied with a work-out on the barbell – commencing sometimes with the empty shaft weighing 55 lb. ("Berg" pattern). Starting with a One-hand Snatch and going on to One-Hand Cleaning and Pressing. He would work up with the weight increasing on the bar to a point when he would switch to Two-hands Snatching and then on to Cleaning and Jerking. Usually, the bar would finish with the top men of the Club Jerking 308 lb., and, after all were through for the night, Hermann would go on and have the bar made up to 319.5, 330.5, 352.5 lb., which he would proceed to Clean and Jerk – sometimes with ordinary grip, sometimes with reverse grip. He would do his Two-Hands Snatching and Jerking occasionally with the feet remaining together throughout the lift – giving only slightly at the knees. In this manner he would work up to 330.5 lb. on the Jerk. A further training feat of Hermann's was to Clean and Jerk the barbell of 330.5 lb. overhead and then hold it there whilst he took away one leg to the side – he would swing this out to the side and then back, immediately transferring the weight over to that leg and swinging out to the side the opposite leg. Starting with a slow tempo, he would speed it up until he was almost hopping on alternate legs swinging the opposing leg to the side – with the barbell held overhead throughout! At other times Hermann would hold the weight overhead and then unlock his arms and lower the weight a few inches, immediately pressing it out and relocking his arms – repeating this movement for several repetitions. He would also practise Cleaning a weight for five to six repetitions and then Jerk it overhead after the sixth Clean. In this manner, he would work up from 275.5 lb. to 286.5 lb. Then take 308.5 lb. for three "Cleans" and one final Jerk. Two "Cleans" with 330.5 lb. and one Jerk. Sometimes he would round out this session by performing Upright Rowing Motions of two to three repetitions with the barbell, ranging from 220.5 lb. 242.5 lb. and 253.5 lb.

Thus might end a typical work-out covering two hours – working fast all the while and not pausing to "natter" during his training session. Hermann did his talking and discussing after his work-out was over for the day.

On other evening training sessions he might, after working through The Chain, perform some Curls, Presses and Holdouts with both one and two hands, whilst sitting on the floor. These lifts might be performed with kettlebells, dumb-bells or barbell as the mood took him. In all these lifts he usually performed two repetitions – never more than three – then increased the weight. Sitting on a chair, Hermann would do Swings and Presses, Holdouts and Crucifix and also Curls, from the same position. On other occasions, he might do his regular barbell work-out with different grips, gripping with the hands close together, wide apart, crossed grip, reversed grip and so on. Or he would sit astride a bench and Clean a barbell off the bench, then whilst in this position he would Press or Push the barbell overhead. A further

www..StrongmanBooks.com

variation would be to kneel down on the floor and Clean the bar to the shoulders from this position. There were, to be exact, two positions on the knees – one kneeling upright on the knees and the second kneeling and letting the buttocks rest on the heels – both positions were used in training by Hermann.

In the Görner Club at Leipzig there were usually three barbells and lifting platforms in constant use. No. 1 was for the beginners, the barbell usually being between 100 to 150 lb. in weight. No. 2 was for the experienced lifters, the barbell here being mostly 150 to 200 lb., whilst No. 3 platform was where the heavy Dead Lifts and Deep Knee Bends were performed with a barbell usually loaded to 300- or 400 to 500 lb. Depending on his energy on any given training evening, Hermann would start at any one of these platforms with whatever weight happened to be on the bar at that moment. At other times, as I have said, he would commence with the shaft of the bar only.

Training for Special Feats

(i) The Dead Lifts – Training for One-Hand Dead Lifting

For creating a record or attempting to break a record in One- or Two-Handed Dead Lifts, Görner usually trained for two to three weeks before the attempt, getting in either six or nine training sessions – occasionally more, sometimes less. Hermann did not like repetitions in Dead Lifting, but would practise the lift in some variations, increasing the weight by 10 or 15 kilos (22 and 33 lb.). Very rarely would he increase his further attempts by 20 kilos (44 lb.). When using low poundages (for him) in the One- and Two-hands Dead Lifts, Görner would sometimes lower the bar from the finishing position back down to the floor, and, *without touching the floor*, he would again lift the bar back into the finishing position. When practising the One-hand Dead Lifts with low poundages, Görner would sometimes keep his disengaged arm held out at shoulder-level sideways throughout the lift, instead of gaining support from it by placing the non-lifting arm on the corresponding leg and pressing downwards, as is more usual in this lift.

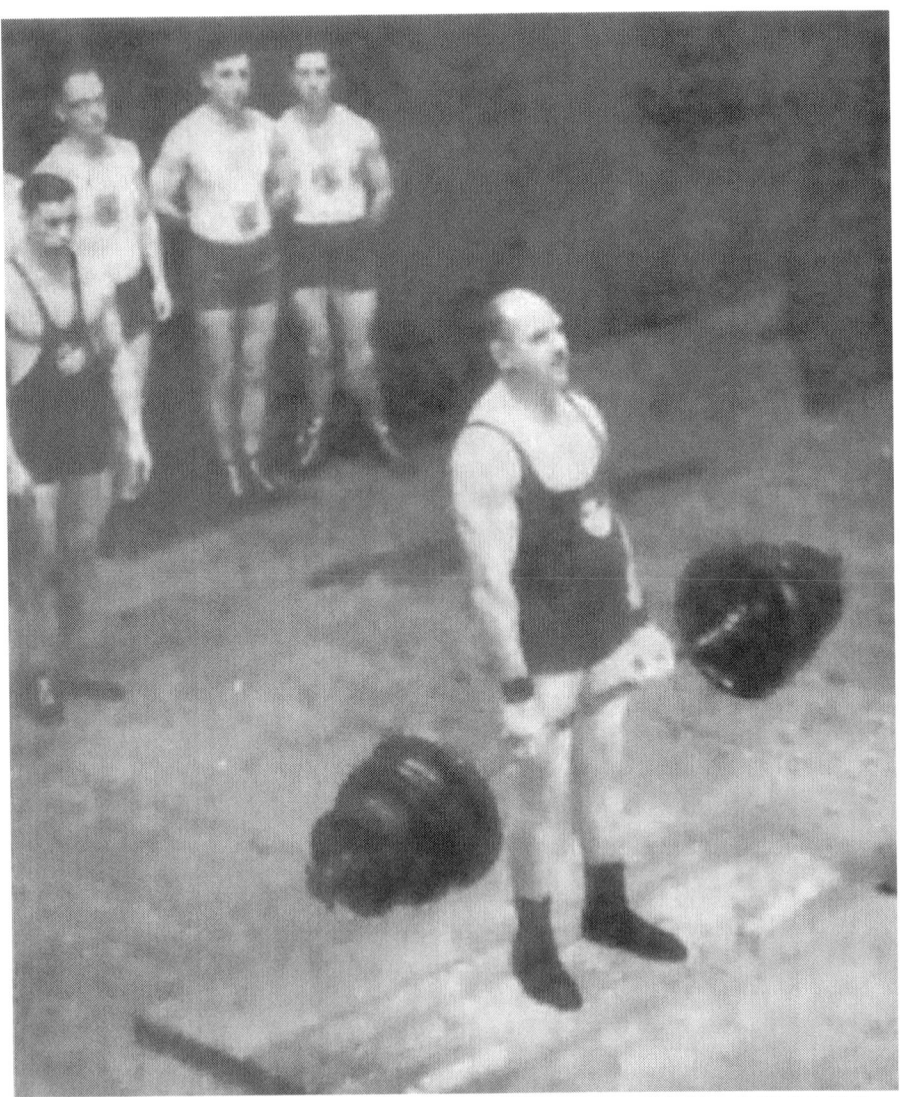

Hermann Görner demonstrating a four-finger Dead Lift of 595 1/2 lb. (270 kilos), using only the index and middle fingers of each hand. Performed on 30th November, 1933, at Leipzig.

Naturally, when making his Record attempts he used the disengaged hand in this fashion. Hermann practised all his Dead Lifts on straight bars with regular plates, using mostly the Berg-type and sometimes the Schwedler-type revolving barbell. At no time was the bar higher from the floor than 8.25 inches (21 cms.). I list hereunder his method of training for One-hand Dead Lifts and will describe in detail the various grips he used for strengthening his fingers and grip.

For One-hand Dead Lifts with the barbell parallel with the lifter's front, the following variation of grip would be used equally over two training sessions, making usually three lifts with each grip – very rarely would he perform four attempts.

Grip No. 1

One-hand Dead Lift using thumbless overhand grip with four fingers only. In this style, Hermann would lift the bar by gripping it in the *first* joint of his fingers – the hand was *not* closed so that the ends of the fingers touched the palm. In other words, the fingers were at full stretch except the first joint which encircled the barbell shaft – the thumb was kept quite clear of the bar throughout. In this style he would do 220.5 lb., 253.5 lb., 275.5 lb., and has lifted 330.75 lb. as a maximum.

Grip No. 2

One-hand Dead Lift using thumbless overhead grip – the more usual style of thumbless grip. The fingers were wrapped round the shaft of the barbell and touched his palm, as the whole of the hand was closed – the thumb placed on the shaft the same side as the fingers. For lifting in this manner, he took the following poundages: – 330.75 lb., 363.75 lb., and 385.75 lb. As a maximum, he has lifted 463 lb.

Grip No. 3

One-hand Dead Lift using normal overhand grip – the usual grip with the thumb going round the shaft in the opposite direction to the fingers. Using 3 attempts again, he lifted the following poundages: – 463, 485, 507 lb. As a maximum, he has lifted in this manner 554.48 lb., also on a non-revolving Domke straight bar.

Grip No. 4

One-hand Dead Lift with Bent Arm with over-hand hook grip. In this fashion, the lifting arm was half-bent at the elbow and *kept in this position* throughout the lift. The grip used was the normal overhand grip *with hook* and the bar lifted from floor to waist-level. In this style Hermann would do – again one attempt with each poundage – 242.5, 264.5 and 286.5 lb. He has lifted 330.75 lb. in this style.

Grip No. 5

One-hand Dead Lift, in rapid Half Snatching motion, using overhand hook grip. In this style, the bar was lifted in succession as quickly as possible, taking the following poundages: – 396.75, 418.75, 441 lb. In this manner Hermann has handled 499.36 lb. on a straight Domke bar, which is not a revolving type.

Grip No.6

One-hand Dead Lift using overhand hook grip and heavy poundages. Hermann here would take the following poundages in his training: – 529, 551.25, 617.25, 661.25 lb. His maximum lift in this style being 727.5 lb. as listed in his Records.

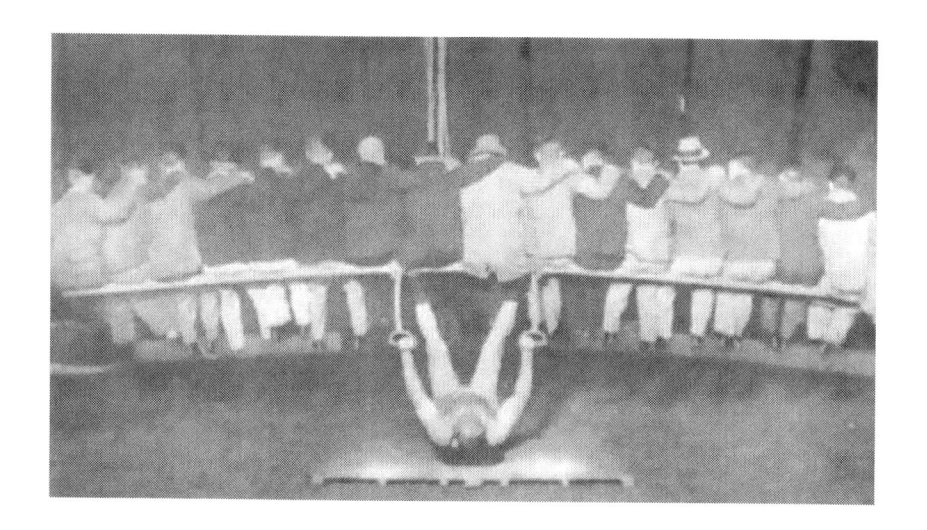

The famous "Plank" feat as performed by Görner. He is here shown supporting over 2,500 lb. Photograph taken in South Africa whilst touring with Pagel's Circus.

GOERNER THE MIGHTY

(ii) TRAINING FOR TWO-HAND DEAD LIFTING

Görner usually took one lift with each poundage and would take his lifts in four of the under-listed styles at each training session – or to put it another way – it would take him three work-outs to go through the 12 variations of gripping listed below, taking at each work-out 4 of these variations. Particularly noted should be the great attention Hermann gave to strengthening his fingers and gripping-powers by working out in this thorough fashion. Now I will list his methods of training for his enormous Two-handed Dead Lifts.

Grip No. 1

Two-finger Dead Lift using only the index fingers with an overhand grip. In this manner Hermann merely used the index finger of each hand. The barbell would weight : – 132.25 lb., 157.25 lb., 176.25 lb. or similar. One attempt with each poundage. He has lifted 187.5 lb. in this manner, but it did not represent his limit.

Grip No. 2

Two-finger Dead Lift using index fingers and reverse grip. One-finger lifting in overhand and one finger in underhand grip in other words. In this manner, weights of 176.25 lb., 220.5 lb. and 264.5 lb. or similar were used. He has lifted 286.5 lb. in this style – nowhere near his maximum.

Grip No. 3

Two-finger Dead Lift using only the middle fingers of each hand – normal overhand grip. He would take the following poundages : – 154.25 lb., 176.25 lb., 198.5 lb. He has lifted 220.5 lb. in this manner – again well under his maximum.

Grip No. 4

Two-finger Dead Lift using only middle fingers and a reverse grip – similar to Grip No. 2 – lifting 198.5 lb., 242.5 lb. and 286.5 lb. or similar. He has lifted 308.75 lb. in this manner.

www..StrongmanBooks.com

Grip No. 5

Four-finger Dead Lift using only the index and middle fingers and an overhand grip. Lifting 286.5 lb., 308.75 lb., and 330.75 lb. Görner has lifted 385.75 lb. in this style – again not his limit.

Grip No. 6

Four-finger Dead Lift using only index and middle fingers with reverse grip. Poundages of 463, 507, 551.25 lb. for no more than one attempt with each. He has lifted 595.75 lb. in this manner but not his limit by any means.

Measurements of a Brick

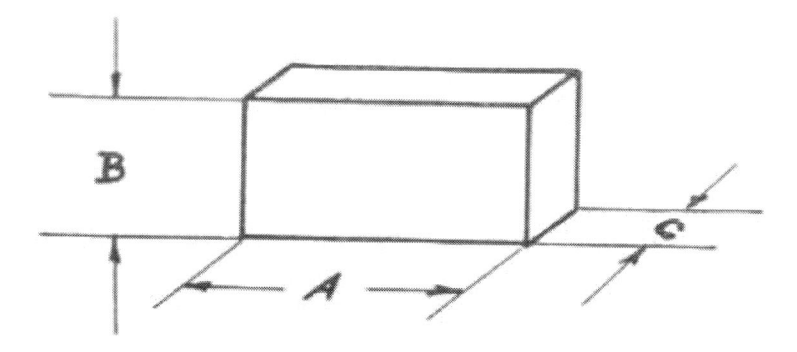

A = Length, 10 ¼ in. or 26 cm.

B = Height 5 1/8 in. or 13 cm.

C = Width, 2 5/16 in. or 6.5 cm.

Average Weight = 4 kilos or 8.82 lb.

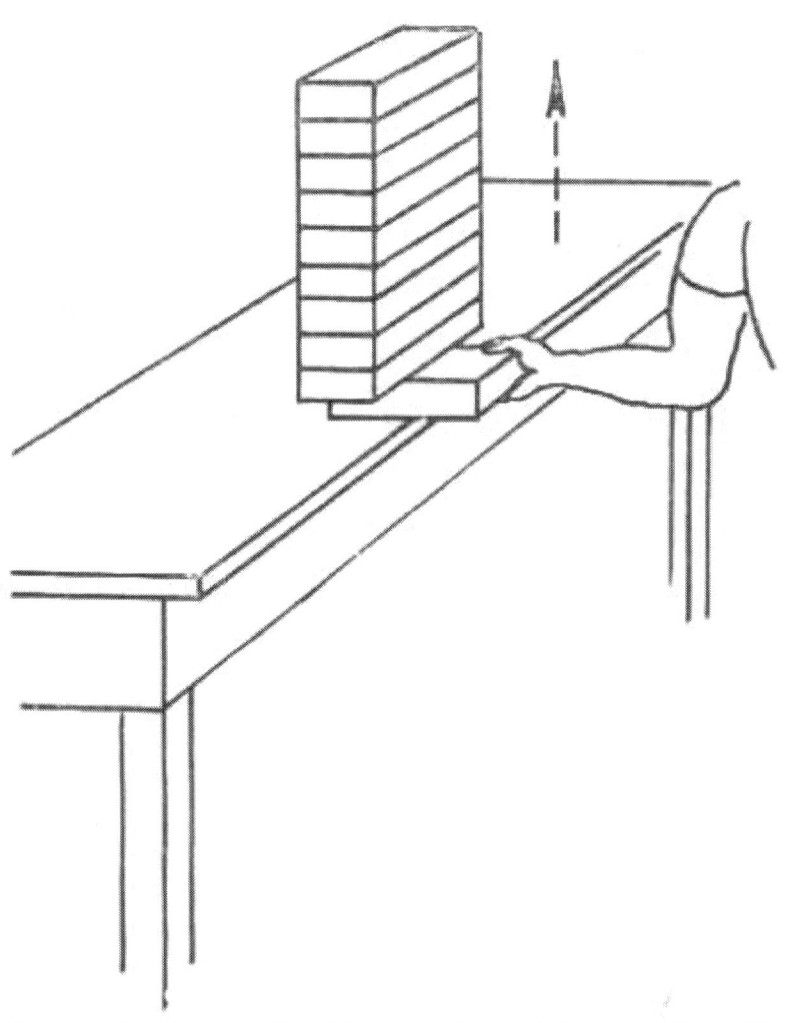

Picking up with the right hand from a table to bricks totalling 88¼ lb. (40 kilos) in weight. Lifted with the palm upwards with the thumb above, the arm remained half-bent, as shewn in the sketch, throughout the lift.

Grip No. 7

Two-hands Dead Lift using normal overhead grip without hooking: – 595.25 lb., 628.25 lb., and 661.25 lb., one attempt with each poundage. Maximum lift here was 727.5 lb.

Grip No. 8

Two-hands Stiff-legged Dead Lift using normal overhand grip without hooking. Poundages of 551.25, 573.25, and 595.25, each lifted once. Has lifted 661.25 lb. in this manner.

Grip No. 9

Two-hands Rapid Dead Lift using overhand hook grip. Taking one attempt for each poundage, Hermann would handle 441 lb., 474 lb., and 507 lb. He has lifted 554.48 lb. in this fashion – the weight being lifted to waist-level! He started this lift with straight arms and then bent his arms as his terrific "pull" took the bar to waist-height.

Grip No. 10

Two-hands Bent-arm Dead Lift using overhand hook grip. In this style, the arms remained bent half-way through the entire lift. The weight was lifted to waist-level. Poundages : – 330.75 lb., 363.75 lb., 396.75 lb. In this manner Hermann has lifted 441 lb., but he could have done more.

Grip No. 11

Two-hands Dead Lift with heavy weights, using either overhand hook grip or reverse grip, taking the following poundages with one lift on each : – 639.25 lb., 683.5 lb. and 727.5 lb. His maximum lifts using overhand hook grip were 793.75 lb. (barbell only) and, with reverse grip, 830 lb. (barbell plus two men standing on it).

Grip No. 12

Two-barbells Dead Lift. Using two barbells and standing between them using overhand grip with hook. Weight of both bells (combined) would be: 529 lb., 551.25 lb. and 573.25 lb. Hermann has lifted in this manner 617.25 lb. officially and 663.5 lb. unofficially (right arm 332.75 lb. and left arm 330.75 lb.), which he lifted and walked with for 23 feet across the training-hall in Leipzig on 10th September, 1920.

That describes Hermann Görner's methods of training for his enormous Dead Lifts. In addition to the training described above, Hermann would also practise the following lifts, doing in the "Bend-over" one lift with each poundage and in the "Shrugging" 4 to 6 repetitions in succession.

Bendover with Barbell across shoulders

Also known as the "Good Morning" exercise. Keeping the legs straight and bending until the body was parallel to the floor, he would take the following poundages: – 220.5 lb., 242.5 lb., 264.5 lb. He has performed this lift with a barbell of 335.87 lb., which was done in Leipzig in 1932.

Shoulder-shrugging with barbell

Holding the barbell in front of his thighs, Hermann would take 683.5 lb., 716.5 lb., 749.5 lbs. His maximum lift in this manner was 2 repetitions with 852 lb. – using a reverse grip and lifting the bar plus two men, Hermann took it in the "hang" position and from there "shrugged" it twice!

Shoulder-shrugging combined with Arm-shrugging

The title of this may sound a little strange, but I cannot think of how to describe it differently! In this feat the shoulders were shrugged in the usual manner and the arms were also bent or "shrugged" about 3 to 4 in. at the same time – I hope my readers can follow my description. In this fashion, Hermann used 573.25 lb., 595.25 lb. and 617.25 lb. As a maximum lift, he has done three repetitions with 719.8 lb. using a reverse grip with hook. The barbell was handed to him at the "hang" position, from where Hermann "shrugged" it! Bending the arms also at the same time.

Arm-shrugging without shoulder shrugging

Holding the barbell in the finishing position of the Two-hands Dead

Lift, Hermann would then lift it about 4 in. by bending his arms slightly at the elbows – "shrugging" his arms in other words. His shoulders were, however, kept in normal position and not shrugged as well. In this manner he handled weights of 418.75 lb., 441 lb., and 463 lb. One of his best lifts in this manner was 6 repetitions with 554.48 lb., which he did with thumbless overhand grip only on fingertips on a non-revolving bar – this was in 1931, in Leipzig.

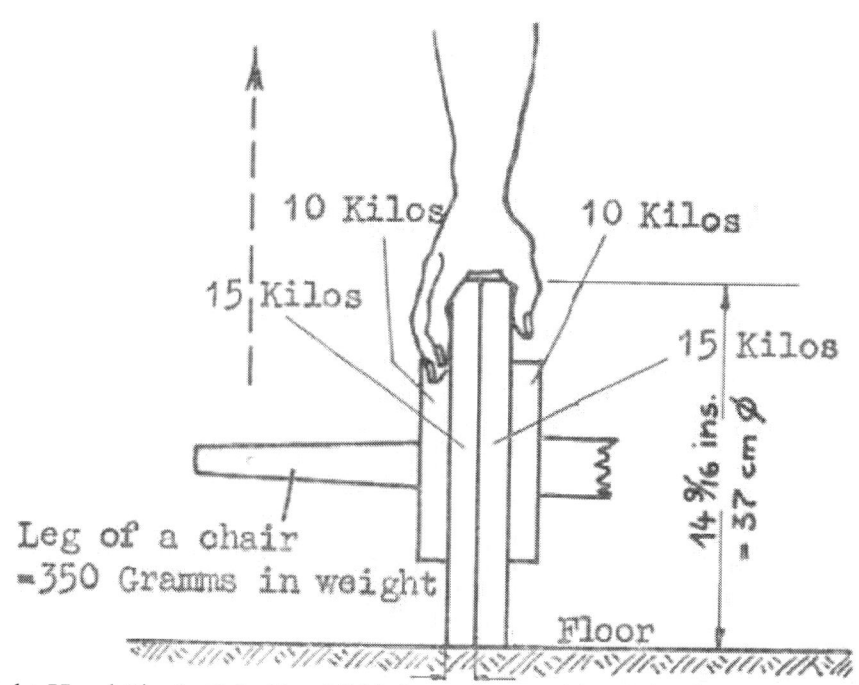

Right-Hand Pinch-Grip Dead Lift from the outside of the foot of 111 lb. (50.35 kilos) on 2 3/8 in. (60 mm.) thick object correctly picked up to the dead-hang by Hermann GÖRNER on July 10th, 1934, at LEIPZIG.

GOERNER THE MIGHTY

(iii) TRAINING FOR SUPPORTING OR CARRYING FEATS

The equipment used by most of the members of the Leipzig Athletic Club for supporting or carrying feats consisted of two similar pieces of apparatus. The smaller one of these consisted of a bar 200 to 225 cm. in length (about 6 ft. 7 in. to 7 ft. 4¾ in.), 48 to 50 cm. (about 2 in.) in diameter. At each end of the bar was attached a short length of strong chain, and a second short length of chain was also fastened about 24 inches distance from each end of the bar. To the ends of these two chains (four in all – two each end of the bar), a short length of rod or piping was fastened and thus a man could sit at each end of the bar, placing himself on the short length of rod attached by the chains to the long bar and balancing himself by holding the long bar with his hands. I think my readers will be able to follow my description. This piece of apparatus would hold two-men – one at either end – and was usually used for handwork in supporting feats. The second piece of equipment was exactly similar to the first except that it was longer by about 10 inches and the shorter rods were also longer to permit of two men sitting side by side on the lower bar. This was generally used for legwork. Both pieces of apparatus were used for supporting and carrying work when the bars would be used across the shoulders of the performer.

For supporting on the feet several men, a large plank was used. This was from between 4 to 6 metres. long (a metre is 39.37 in.) with a width of 20 to 25 cm. (about 8 to 10 in.) and 2¾ in. to 3¼ in. thick. The plank was placed on top of two trestles – one at either end – the height of these being about 100 to 115 cm. (39.37 in. to 45 in. approx.). To train with this plank, the lifter would take up his position on his back on the floor – using a specially constructed back-rest which was padded for comfort – then two men would sit upon the plank, which would then be pressed up off the trestles about 2 to 4 in. and supported for several seconds on the feet of the performer. After some practice at this, the load would be pressed up by the feet and the two trestles would be quickly removed by assistants. Sometimes beneath the plank would be iron hand-grips screwed to it. These hand-grips would be gripped by the performer and used by him for balancing purposes only – they were not used for pressing or supporting the plank. Some planks had handles screwed underneath, something like the handles of kettle-bells – these were used in similar manner for balancing purposes only. The modern "Leg-Press" machines were not known in Germany and most Leg Presses were done with the "Sitting-Bars" or with barbells.

When Hermann Görner started in his youth to train for supporting loads upon his feet he began by pressing, whilst lying on his back, the empty two-man or 4-man sitting bars; after getting the hang of this, he started with Leg Presses with the same apparatus, doing only low repetitions. After perfecting this, he then trained supporting 2 to 5 men upon his feet – using the sitting-bar apparatus I have described. Then he would bend his knees slightly and press the whole load up again. When perfect in this style, he started supporting weights at the same time in his hands – at first with a barbell which he would press overhead whilst holding the weight of 2 to 5 men on his feet – he would press the bar out, then lower it slightly and press up again. Later, when he had perfected his performance in this style, Hermann practised the so-called "Tomb of Hercules". That is, whilst lying on his back he would support a load upon his feet and hands simultaneously. In Germany this feat was known as "The Pyramid", and in this fashion Hermann has supported 2 barbells and no fewer than 8 men!

"The Plank" feat was practised in a similar fashion. At first the empty plank, then 2 men, and then as his strength increased with practice so would the number of men on the plank be increased until he would be holding up 16 or more men. He has, in fact, held up as many as 24 men, as is described in another chapter of this book.

For strengthening his legs and back, Hermann would take a barbell plus 4 men sitting on it, across his shoulders – sometimes a fifth man would sit astride his shoulders – and with this load he would make some half-squats or knee-bends: no wonder he developed strong legs!

The so-called "Caroussel" or "Merry-Go-Round", or turning around on his own axis with a barbell and men hanging on it supported across his shoulders, Görner would practise with a barbell and 5 or 6 men, sometimes 7 men, quickly turning round 5, 6 or 7 times, or he would sometimes vary this by walking several steps with the load. This feat is particularly good training for carrying heavy loads. Another similar feat was the supporting of very heavy weights across the shoulders. This was performed by Hermann with a barbell and eleven men! Five men would hang on each end of the bar and the eleventh would sit astride his shoulders. Usually, however, he would train upon his feat with 8 or 9 men – 4 at each end of the bar and the ninth man upon his shoulders. Through the practice of this feat, Görner developed an enormous vertebral bone in the neck region which reached the dimensions of a boy's fist – this enormous bone can be felt by anyone meeting Görner to-day – I have never come across its like in any other strong man. When my friend Alfred Schrader and myself felt this bone formation we wondered how any man could possess such enormous bone structure. Hermann would smile on these occasions and say that his bone was built to that size and form by jerking a barbell from behind his neck and then allowing the bar to drop back onto his neck! On 21st December, 1931, we saw him take a barbell of 330.75 lb., Clean and Jerk it and then allow it to drop from arms' length to the back of his neck – the bar which was 1 3/16 in. in diameter immediately became a "cambered" bar!

(iv) TRAINING FOR A MATCH

When Görner was an amateur he would train for a match for 3 to 4 weeks before the match took place, usually 3 training sessions per week, each one consisting of 2 hours' work-out. In Görner's youth the matches were usually made upon 5 lifts – One-hand Snatch, One-hand Clean and Jerk (performed sometimes with the opposite hand), and the Three Olympics – Two-hands Press, Snatch and Clean and Jerk.

For each lift, he would do 3 or sometimes 4 repetitions and then increase the weight, usually going up in stages of 5 kilos (10 lb.). Beginning with the Right-hand he would go on to the Left-hand with his Snatches and Jerks before proceeding to the double-handed lifts. For both One-handed and Two-handed Snatching, Hermann would train by snatching the barbell from the "hang" and also by taking the barbell off two chairs. It should be stressed that Hermann favoured low repetitions – usually 3 and very rarely 4 – with the weight being increased by 5 kilos (10 lb.) after each set. He trained for quality of muscle as opposed to quantity – that he also got quantity in the process was, as far as he was concerned, purely coincidental! He was interested in training for strength; first and foremost in his mind was the ability to do things with his muscles, not just to have large muscles which were pretty to look upon, but when put to the test fell down. The training that Hermann did saw to it that, his muscles, whilst being developed, were also developed with the highest-quality tissue – they were not blown up by endless repetitions with light weights. In that fashion, Hermann avers a man can never become strong – really strong – he *must* lift heavy weights, and the weights *must* be increased as his strength grows: this is the *only* way to become a strong man.

Additional Training Information

Under this heading, I propose to list briefly Görner's views on other important aspects of training. To begin with what is one of the most important: –

(i) *Diet*

Görner is firmly convinced that a mixed diet is the best for a strong man, with emphasis laid on eating good meals with the accent on meat! He is particularly partial to pork and beef and also wurst – German sausagemeat. Vegetables also, together with potatoes, but not overdoing the latter. He is very fond of nuts – particularly walnuts – and all fruits: apples especially, which he thinks every strong man should eat, as well as oranges and other citrous fruits. Cheese and eggs also figure in his diet, but he does not care for rich pastries nor does he drink milk in any quantity. As regards drinking, he drinks beer, but only moderately – seldom touches spirits – and was a non-smoker until his twenties and afterwards only a moderate smoker.

(ii) *Massage*

Görner holds the opinion that massage is not so very important for weight lifters. He has used massage only on rare occasions – to ease

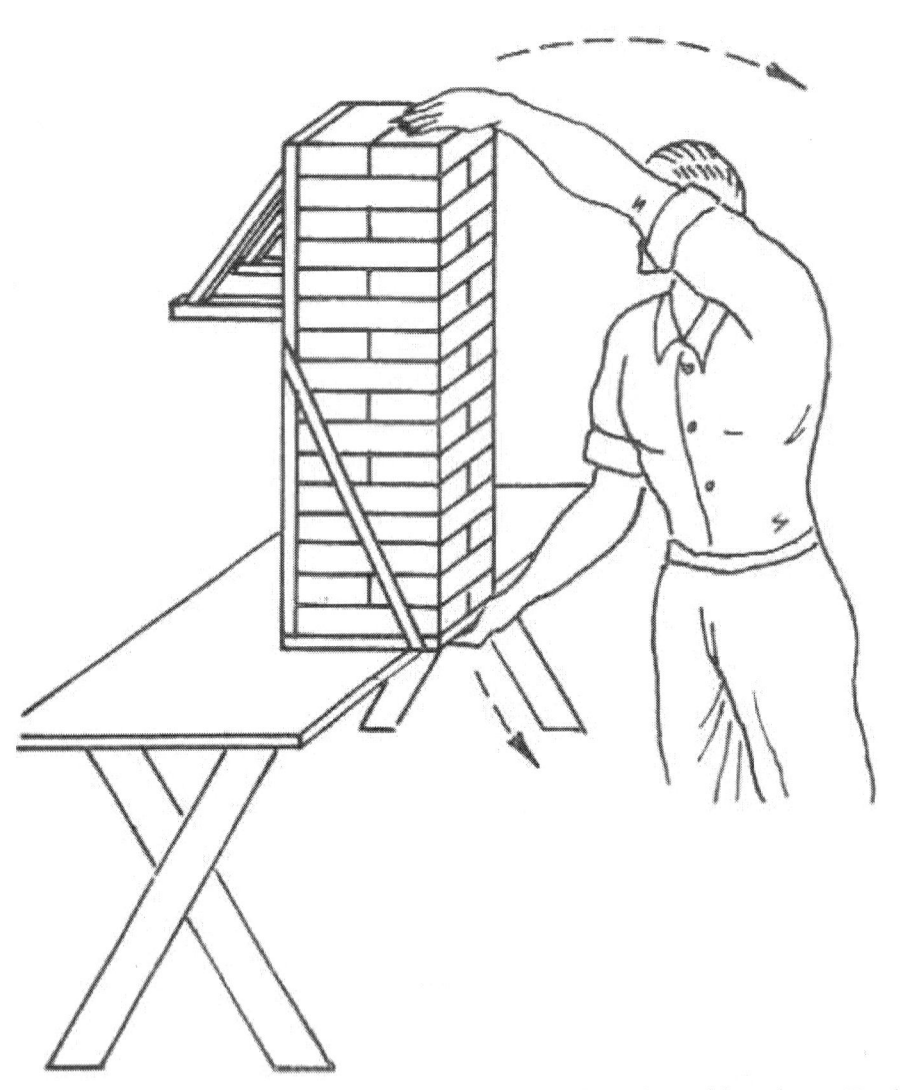

Lifting 32 bricks simultaneously from a bench and stacking them. Each pile totalled 282 ¼ lb. (128 kilos) in weight. This feat was performed continuously for eight hours per day!

a strain or undue stiffness, but in general it is his opinion that massage is most useful when a man suffers from poor circulation, and most weight lifters have excellent circulation. So his advice is to take massage sparingly – find out for yourself if it is of benefit and decide accordingly.

(iii) *Roadwork*

Görner has always performed a certain amount of roadwork in his training. Usually a thirty-minute jog-trot and walk combined, twice weekly – mostly before doing his open-air training in the summer months in the Germania Bath as I have described.

(iv) *Sunbathing*

It is the opinion of Hermann Görner that excessive sunbathing or getting a heavy tan can be overdone. He would train in the open air and in the process get a light tan, but he is of the opinion that excessive sunbathing is detrimental and not necessary for super-health. Again, it is largely a matter of personal choice, but it is Hermann's opinion that sunbathing is greatly over-rated as being necessary for a strong man.

(v) *Swimming*

This, he considers, every man should indulge in – and mix with open-air weight training. I have referred to his methods already, so will not repeat myself.

(vi) *Sleep*

Here Hermann considers a strong man should always obtain sufficient sleep to repair the demands he has made upon his system. He advocates eight to nine hours' regular sleep, and in his own case would usually take a nap of about an hour after lunch each day when engagements permitted.

(vii) *Sex*

Moderation should be the keynote in the sexual habits of strongmen. One cannot develop into an outstanding strongman and continually indulge in sexual excesses. Görner has always been an abstemious man in this respect and he considers it essential to the successful development of outstanding strength, that one observes moderation in sexual indulgence.

In this chapter I have outlined the methods which were used so successfully in developing Hermann Görner's enormous strength, and it is hoped that his methods and training habits may prove of help in assisting would-be strongmen to reach their goal – that of becoming strong with a capital "S"! If carefully studied and assiduously put into practice, I am quite sure these methods will help the serious strength student as much as they have helped many hundreds of other men in Germany and elsewhere in the past.

EDGAR MÜLLER

CHAPTER 7

His Attitude to Lifting and Feats of Strength

I HAVE been an actual eye witness of 75% of Hermann Görner's best feats of strength. I have personally judged, checked and recorded nearly 1,400 public lifts and feats of strength performed by this wonderful superman. The feats, lifts and stunts have been as varied as the ingenuity of Hermann could devise. Hermann made no rehearsal of his feats – in the majority of cases these were impromptu and gave no indication of his maximum powers.

Authorities other than myself have unanimously agreed that his gigantic strength has never been plumbed and that had he had the ambition to specialize or to go into disciplined training, he would have established records that would have stood for all time. It should be noted that many of his best feats were actually accomplished after the age of 40. At the age of 43, he created world records in weight lifting.

"My health is more important than a record," he would retort, when zealous fans would advise him to go after records. He lifted for the sheer pleasure of testing his super-human powers.

"Variety is the spice of life," declared Hermann. He was an all-round strong man and had no love for the monotonous 'Olympic Three' as the be-all and end-all of the lifter. Görner practised all lifts, including very many that are not in the book, but he did not favour the Bent Press, which he considered a 'trick lift', adapted for long-trunked and short-legged men, who can very easily bend far to the side. He also frowned on 'expander' exercises, believing that such forms of exercise destroyed the explosive force needed in performing quick lifts. Teeth lifting he considered a most unnatural method of showing one's strength. A 'nonsense' feat to use his own expression!

Görner has never received training or any formal instruction from anyone other than himself. His methods were simply of his own devising. Right from his very inception to the world of Strength in 1905, he trained himself and showed others that he had the goods and a

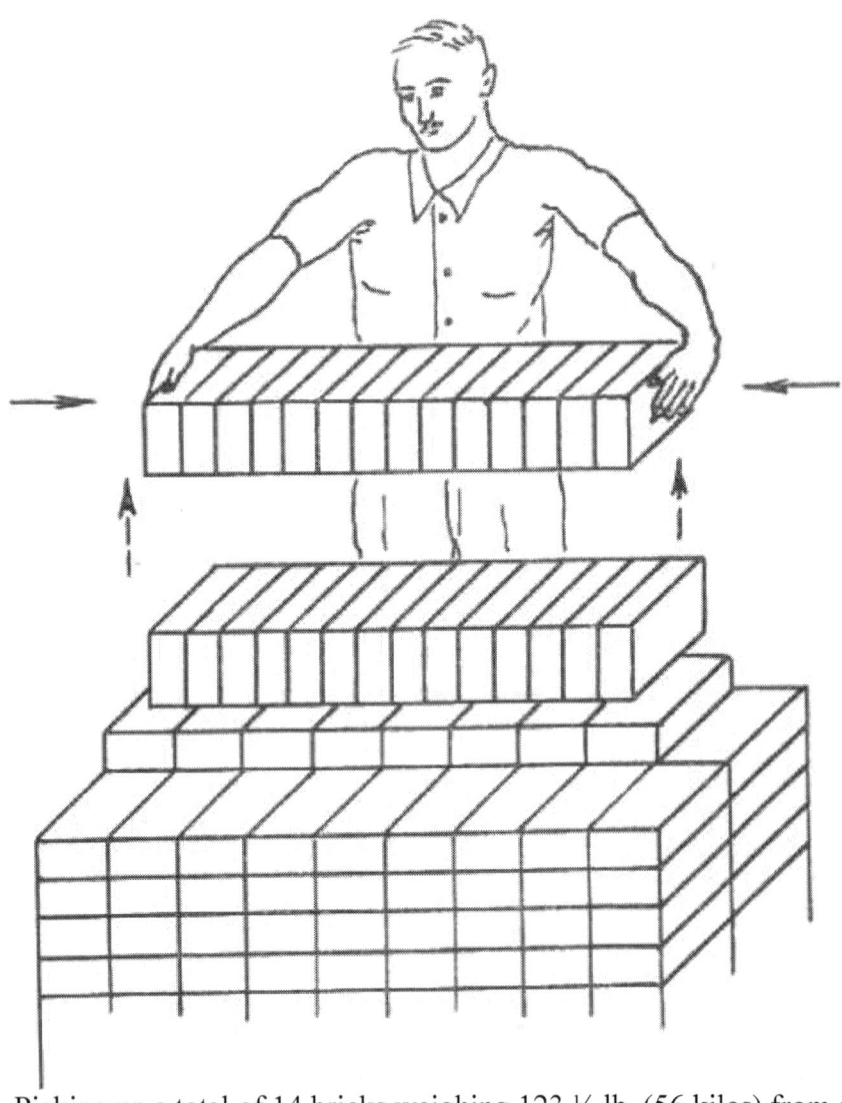

Picking up a total of 14 bricks weighing 123 ½ lb. (56 kilos) from a stack. The bricks were lifted by being squeezed together – at no time were the upper arms or bricks in contact with the body.

most efficacious system to bring about such a happy state of affairs.

At the lifting of kettleweights, Hermann was certainly the world's best exponent. Dumb-bells also took up a considerable amount of his training time, as well as the more orthodox feats performed with the barbell. He was a great believer in mixing slow movements with weights, such as Curls and Presses in with faster Jerks and Snatches, in order to create all-round lifting efficiency.

As a proof of his agility, notwithstanding his great body-weight, Hermann has performed a standing high jump, with heels together, over a chair of 32 in. high. He has also made a standing broad jump of 10 ft. 4 in. at a time when he weighed over 20 stone. The best proof of Görner's incomparable strength and sheer bodily power can be gauged by his stupendous performances on the double and single-handed dead lifts. Hermann's method of performing the dead lifts was the hardest way. There was no resting of the bell on the thighs above the knees or shifting of the grips. Just one mighty pull only and he stood erect and held the weight for more than the required period.

His records were almost without exception performed 'cold', without any preliminary 'warming up' with lighter weights. Very few people are aware that he actually performed the colossal feat of a One-hand Dead Lift of 727 ½ lb. on a Berg revolving barbell, on 8th October, 1920, at Leipzig. On the same Berg barbell – which was, of course, a straight bar and not a cambered one – he did his Two-hands Dead Lift of 793 ¾ lb., twenty-one days later. This stupendous weight was held for five seconds in the finishing position. As a witness of this feat, I will remember the frantic enthusiasm of his audience and the smiling and unruffled acknowledgment of Hermann. After a few minutes' pause, Görner asked for 300 kilos (661 lb.) to be put on the bar with which he proposed to perform a Right-hand Dead Lift. At the first attempt he lifted the bar parallel to his front with the right hand correctly, to the unanimous approval of the judges, fixing and holding it in the finishing position for four seconds. On weighing the bell, it was found to turn the scales at 301 kilos, i.e., 663½ lb. This feat received thunderous applause from his audience. As a matter of interest, his body-weight at the time was 220½ lb. (100 kilos).

Certain writings outside of Germany have carried many garbled reports on Hermann's extraordinary Dead Lifting ability. Calculated it would seem to reflect unfavourably on the appliances used. One writer has claimed that Görner used a 10 ft. bar specially made for the occasion with, it was alleged, slotted discs. The ignorance of the writers of these statements is more to be pitied than condemed. It may be stated quite categorically that in all his Dead Lifts Hermann Görner used the well-known Berg 'Hantel' with ordinary discs and straight bar. I would like to go on record as saying that long special bars with slotted plates were unknown in any of the Clubs where Hermann lifted, although I understand that barbells with such plates or similar were used in Dead Lifts by some lifters in other parts of Europe.

I respect the great feats of the famous French lifters, Rigoulot and Cadine, but their best performances on the Dead Lifts, both double and single-handed, can hardly be compared with the lifts of Görner. Rigoulot's best Two-hands Dead Lift was 621¾ lb. and his Right-hand Dead Lift, 450 lb. Cadine's best was 617¼ two hands, with a Single-handed Dead Lift of 449¾ lb.

My own conviction is that had Hermann Görner ever had serious competition from other Strong Men, he would have been inspired to accomplish a Two-hands Dead Lift not far short of the enormous weight of 900 lb.

In 1921 Hermann sustained a knee injury which permanently affected his maximum poundages with such lifts as the Two-hands Dead Lift. Although he was unfamiliar with the British cambered bars, he did do some training in London in W.A. Pullum's Gymnasium, but his best feats in England, although classed as world records, were much behind his records performed earlier in Germany. Surely his stupendous feat performed at the age of 42 on 18th August, 1933, in Leipzig, when he executed a Dead Lift with barbell and human weights totalling 830 lb., gives some indication of his true powers!

What would Hermann have done, when lifting at his best in a contest on the Two-hands Dead Lift in competition with the present day American lifters, Bob Peoples and Bill Boone, can only be left to the imagination. Peoples has lifted the amazing poundage of 725½ lb., whilst weighing only 189 lb. himself. Boone's best Two-hands Lift was around 700 lb. All Hermann's training mates, and I might add myself, knowing Hermann's amazing ability when lifting at his best, hold the firm conviction that, if Görner had specialized in Dead Lifting for such a contest, he would easily have topped 850 lb.

Hermann regarded Dead Lifting and carrying of heavy weights as fundamental tests of bodily strength. Such lifts as hand and thigh lifting, finger lifting, back lifting and harness lifting never interested him. Had it been otherwise, it is my considered opinion that he would have set records that would have stood for all time.

Hermann's hundred and one ways of demonstrating his all-round strength were of such a high order that other 'Kings of Strength', such as Saxon, Steinbach, Swoboda, Cyr, Apollon and Rigoulot, would have found him more than a match for them in an all-round contest. In his Stage and Circus performances, Hermann delighted in devising new ways at demonstrating his stupendous powers. His fertile mind was the originator of many unique and astounding stunts. His deportment before his audiences was one of grace and elegance. All his feats of strength were performed stylishly and easily, his countenance bearing a smile, as he completed his astounding feats of strength.

Hermann possessed amazing forearm and wrist strength, which he demonstrated in no uncertain manner in the sport of 'Wrist Wrestling'. On 17th December, 1934, our hero took on six famous International Professional Wrestlers in Leipzig's Crystal Palace. At this particular time Hermann and myself were judges in the Professional Greaco-Roman Wrestling Contest. The opponents of Hermann in Wrist Wrestling were all well over 6 ft. in height, the tallest of them being no less than 6 ft. 4 ½ in. All six men were beaten by Hermann in just one minute. This was startling tribute to his terrific wrist and forearm strength, as some of the men he beat possessed biceps of over 18 in. In this contest the six men were seated at a table on one side, whilst Hermann occupied the opposite side of the table. Starting with the first man, he rapidly downed his arm and carried on along the row of men until he came to the sixth. As has been already stated, he flattened the forearm of the sixth man before one minute had elapsed. At the finish of this contest Hermann called out smilingly, "Next gentleman, please", but there were no takers. This demonstration of his overwhelming strength left his audience gazing at him in amazement.

One evening, after our usual work-out in the Club, we repaired to our favourite rendezvous, a small restaurant nearby. As the night was cold, the manager requested his wife to bring some more fuel for the stove. This she did and as the manager searched for a hammer with which to break the briquettes, Hermann took the pieces from the hands of the good lady and quite nonchalantly split every one neatly in two by the power of his hands. A total of 15 briquettes, filling a full-sized pail!

On another occasion, an enthusiast asked Hermann, "What can you do in tearing a pack of cards?" "I don't know," came back the reply. Expecting to see Hermann fail, the enthusiast handed him three complete sets of unused German playing cards, plus some additional loose cards – totalling 110 in all. In exactly one second, Hermann's great hands had torn asunder the whole pack of 110 cards!

On occasions, Hermann liked to demonstrate his terrific grip strength. Using the right hand only, he has 'pinch lifted' two 15 kilo plates. These, when placed together, were 2 3/8 in. thick and just over 14 ½ in. in diameter. Through the center hole of the discs was driven a thick leg of a chair, to which an additional 20 kilos was attached. The whole weight altogether was 111 lb. and, using thumb and fingers only, Hermann 'pinch lifted' this from the floor to the hang, holding the weight nonchalantly for several seconds. The sketch on page 102 shows clearly how this lift was made. This was an impromptu feat of strength and at no time has Hermann specialized in 'pinch lifting'.

A feat of arm strength that should be recorded was Hermann's lift which surpassed that of Louis Cyr's stupendous feat of passing over the counter of his bar-room, his tiny wife of 100 lb. seated on his right hand. This lift Hermann bettered in the following manner: After doing a Right Hand Military Press with kettleweight of 110 ¼ lb. (50 kilos) he lowered the weight – which was balanced on his palm – to waist level, and stretching out his right arm he passed it over the table to the

EDGAR MÜLLER

Author, smilingly, with the words, "So, Edgar. Now duplicate it". Performed in Leipzig on 10th July, 1932.

Just before the first World War, when working in the Krupp Ammunition Factory at Essen, Hermann lifted, in a whimsical moment, a shell weighing 784 lb. (355.6 kilos) which he carried and, as a practical joke, placed the huge projectile on the manager's desk, giving that good man the shock of his life. It was some considerable time before the manager was convinced that it had not been deposited there with the aid of a small crane. On another occasion, whilst working in the same factory, Hermann accepted a wager and won it when he took a wheelbarrow, fully loaded with 30 iron castings of a total weight of between 3,100-3,400 lb., and without the assistance of shoulder straps, gripped the shafts of the barrow, stood erect and succeeded in wheeling and balancing this enormous load for the required distance. When touring South Africa from 1924-26 with Pagel's Circus, Hermann's daily wrestle with an elephant used to bring the house down. When he first incorporated this feat into his Act, the elephant was a small bull, weighing 700 lb. (317 ½ kilos). Hermann continued his daily wrestling with the animal up to the time his contract with the Circus expired, many months later, by which time the elephant had grown in weight to no less than 1,500 lb. (680.4 kilos). 'Some' wrestling partner for a mere human weighing 250 lb. odd!

During his stay in England, where Görner was introduced to the British public by the well-known W.A. Pullum, the former 9 stone World's Weight Lifting Champion, Hermann publicly repeated some of his own particular feats. He had lifted greater poundages in Leipzig, when a younger man, but in spite of the toll of the years and his war wounds, the performances are worth recording here for the sake of comparison. Among many lifts the following may be cited: –

151 ½ lb. (68.72 kilos). Right-hand Snatch with barbell. Bar was snatched from two chairs. (Later surpassed with 154 ¼ lb. (70 kilos) on October 2nd, 1931, in Leipzig.)

200 ¾ lb. (91.06 kilos). Right-hand Swing with dumb-bell.

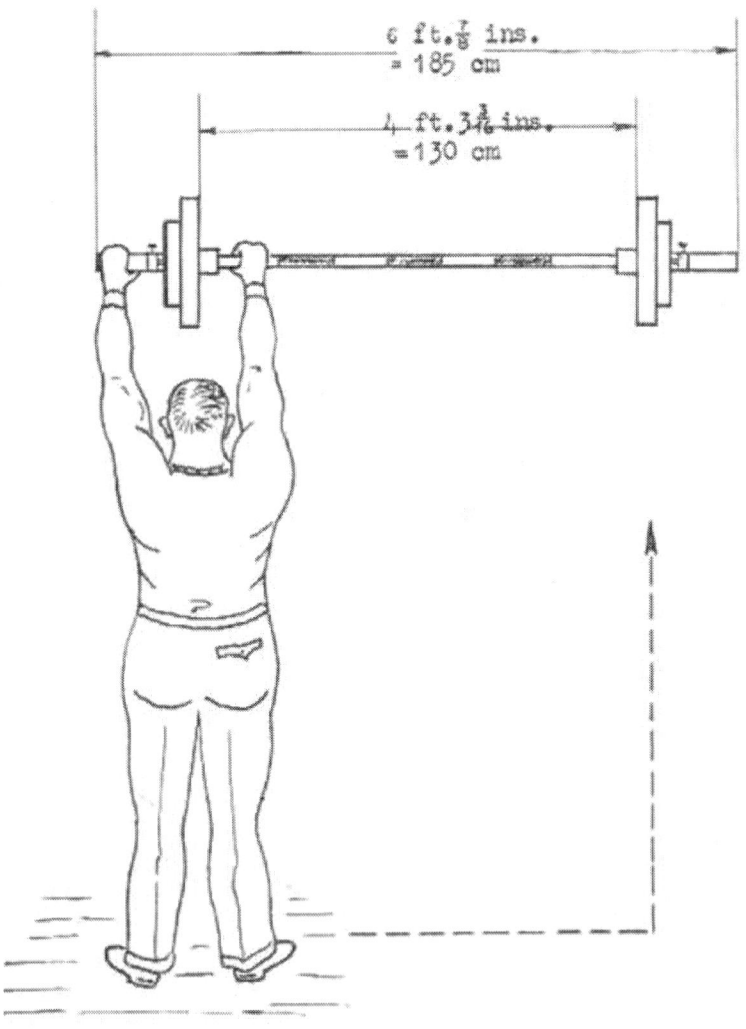

GÖRNER handled a barbell in every possible position. Grasping a barbell of 132¼ lb. (60 kilos) with the left hand over the sleeve – 2 in. in diameter – and with the right hand gripping the shaft tight against the inside collar (closer than shown in sketch), Hermann performed a Two-Hands Snatch from the floor, without moving his feet! Performed on a SCHWEDLER-type revolving barbell, on 27th October, 1931, in LEIPZIG.

EDGAR MÜLLER

224½ lb. (101.8 kilos). Two Dumb-bells Swing. (Surpassed by him with 233¾ lb. (106 kilos) on 25th May, 1933, at Leipzig.)

The above were performed on 16th July, 1927, at Clapham, London, on the occasion of the British 9 Stone Amateur Championships.

279½ lb. (126.7 kilos). Right-hand Clean (only) with barbell. (Görner's best Right-hand Clean was 297 ½ lb. (135 kilos) on November 9th, 1919, in Leipzig.)

302 ¼ lb. (137.1 kilos). Two-hands Clean and Jerk with barbell. In this feat the bar was lifted from two chairs – the stationary 'hang' position – then jerked to arm's length. (This lift was surpassed with 319 ¾ lb. (145 kilos) on November 23rd, 1931, in Leipzig.)

Both the above were performed on 13th August, 1927, at Clapham, London, on the occasion of the 11 Stone British Amateur Championships.

336 ¾ lb. (152 ¾ kilos). Two-hands Clean and Jerk. Jerked twice from the shoulders, once from in front and once from behind the neck. Performed on 2nd July, 1927, at Clapham, on the occasion of the 8 Stone British Amateur Championships.

During his stay in England, Hermann jerked from behind the neck a barbell with human weights making a total of 392 lbs. (177.8 kilos) on 9th August, 1927, at Llanelly; later increased to 411 lb. (186.4 kilos) on 23rd January, 1928, at Oldham. In both of these lifts, the men and the barbell were weighed. Lifting at the famous Camberwell Weight Lifting Club and other London venues, Hermann performed a Right-hand Dead Lift of 602 ¼ lb. (273.18 kilos), a Left-hand Dead Lift of 501 lb. (227 ¼ kilos) and a Two-hands Dead Lift of 652 ¼ lb. (295.86 kilos), the latter lift being performed on 15th March, 1927, at the National Sporting Club. The referee on this occasion being the well-known British Weight Lifting Historian, Writer and Official, W.J. Lowry.

Feat of Abdominal Strength

A barbell weighing 198 ½ lb. (90 kilos) was placed across a bench. Görner sitting astride the same bench first lifted the bar 'clean' with both hands to the shoulders. Then, placing his legs along the bench in the sitting position, he proceeded to press the bar twice overhead – once from the chest and once from behind the neck. Lowering the bar, after the second overhead press, to the chest, Hermann then hooked his feet under the bench (he was still in the sitting position with legs outstretched in front of him) and lowered himself into a supine position still holding the bar in front in the 'clean' position. From the supine position he then came erect – doing a 'sit-up' with 198 ½ lb. held at the chest! This feat of sheer bodily power was performed on 17th November, 1936, when Hermann was 45 years of age.

Grasping an up-ended barbell weighing 230 ¼ lb. (104.5 kilos) with interlaced fingers in the centre, Hermann lifted the bar slowly from the upright position to full arms length overhead, fixing the bar at right angles and holding it for the count. This feat of sheer arm and shoulder strength was performed on 16th February, 1934, at Leipzig.

As a feat of arm and wrist power may be mentioned the following. Hermann first performed an Upright Rowing Motion with a barbell weighing 264 ½ lb. (120 kilos), whilst still holding the bar at shoulder level, he then turned his hands so that the palms faced upwards. The feat was performed by sheer 'wrist' strength on 1st November, 1931, in Leipzig.

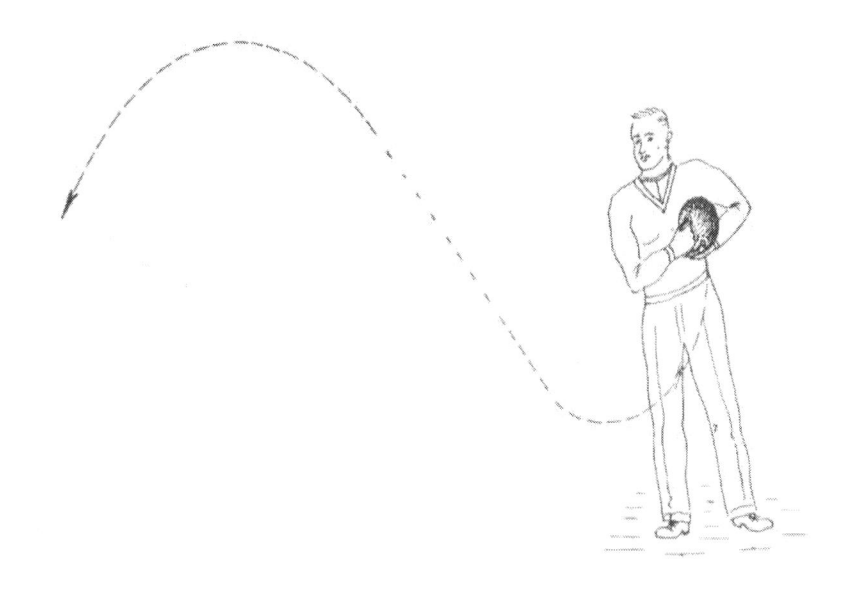

WEIGHT-THROWING

GÖRNER tried a Right-Hand Swing from off the opposite hip with a kettleweight of 132 ¼ lb. (60 kilos), but the weight slipped from his fingers and, through the mighty heave, it flew through the air for exactly 21 feet (6.40 metres), destroying the floor-boards. Performed on 16th April, 1931, at LEIPZIG. GÖRNER then swung the weight right-handed overhead (on the opposite hip) correctly at his second attempt.

For comparison, the late Arthur SAXON is quoted as having swung a 100-lb, kettlebell (also published as 110) from between his legs and then, with a mighty heave, threw it behind his head for a distance of 20 ft. (Date and place, not recorded.)

CONCLUSION

Appreciations by World Famous Authorities

IN order that the reader may gain some idea of the esteem in which Hermann Görner is held by famous authorities and writers on Strong Men and Strength, I propose to give in this chapter extracts and appreciations by many well-known personalities.

Prof. Theodor Siebert of Halle (formerly Alsleben), Germany, one of the leading Continental trainers and still active at the age of 84. It was at Prof. Siebert's Establishment that the famous 'Russian Lion', George Hackenschmidt went to recuperate and train after winning the World's Wrestling Championship in 1901. Prof. Siebert wrote in the *Illustrierter Kraftsport* of 5th February, 1926,

"Hermann Görner, holder of numerous World Records has by his Right-hand Dead Lift of 727 ½ lb. and his Two-hands Dead Lift of 793 ¾ lb., both performed on a regular straight barbell, the greatest right to be acclaimed the strongest man in the world".

The famous American authority, David P. Willoughby, writing in his book *Kings of Arm Strength*, says,

"Hermann Görner was a German professional athlete of extraordinary strength and physique. Standing 6 ft. 1 in. in height and weighing 245lb., his right upper arm measured 18.2 in, his forearm 14.7 in. and his wrist 8.2 in. At his best, Görner weighed 238 lb. in splendid muscular condition, being one of the very few athletes of such weight whose bodies carried no superfluous fat. At this body-weight, his right biceps measured 18 in., his forearm 14.6 in. and his wrist 8.2 in. We shall mention Görner particularly in connection with strength of forearm and grip at which he is pre-eminent. His biceps, however, are, perhaps, unsurpassed for combined size, shape and strength. The only reason we do not cite Görner's feats of pure biceps strength is that such feats have never been published, but he could probably have curled 200 lb. correctly.

[Görner's various feats of arm strength are, of course, revealed in this book, which publishes for the first time the full story of his many amazing strength feats. – *Editors*.]

"It is known that he excelled at every kind of lift where weights are raised to the shoulders. Such lifts, even though using other parts of the body as well, would be sufficient, with the poundages to which Görner was accustomed, to account for the phenomenal development of the 'flexor' muscles of his arms."

Further on in the same book Willoughby writes,

"At this point, it should be sufficient to comment on a subject who is, perhaps, without a peer in feats of this order. We refer to Hermann Görner, the German Strong Man previously cited. No other Strong Man in history has demonstrated an equality with Görner in the lifting of barbells off the ground by strength of grip. In the Right-hand Dead Lift, Görner holds the world's record with 602 ¼ lb. This feat is the greatest single lift on record, being equal in merit to a Two-hands Clean and Jerk of 442 lb.! Görner also holds the record in the Two-hands Dead Lift, having lifted 661.4 lb. (300 kilos) in the French style, a performance that is equivalent to lifting 704 lb. in the English style. The lifting of such poundages from the ground to the erect standing position is indicative of simply colossal strength not only in the grip, but in all parts of the body, particularly the back and legs. It is interesting to note that Görner's hands, unlike those of Marx, are nothing unusual in size. For this reason, his power of grip must be regarded with still greater wonder. In forearm development, Görner certainly leaves nothing to be desired, and although his arm measurements are smaller than those of certain other Heavy Weight Strong Men, it should be remembered that in Görner's case there was no superfluous fat covering the arms."

George F. Jowett of Philadelphia, U.S.A., President of the former American Continental Weight Lifters Association wrote in an article in *Strength* magazine, under the title "Can I name the World's Strongest Man", and said,

"Comparing Görner with other old time and present strong men, such as Steinbach, Swoboda, Rigoulot, etc., I am amazed most by his wonderful lift of 793 ¾ lb. That is an enormous weight to lift off the ground and stand erect. If all the greatest strong men of the world could be brought together, there is no doubt that Hermann Görner would wear the proud title – World's Strongest Man!"

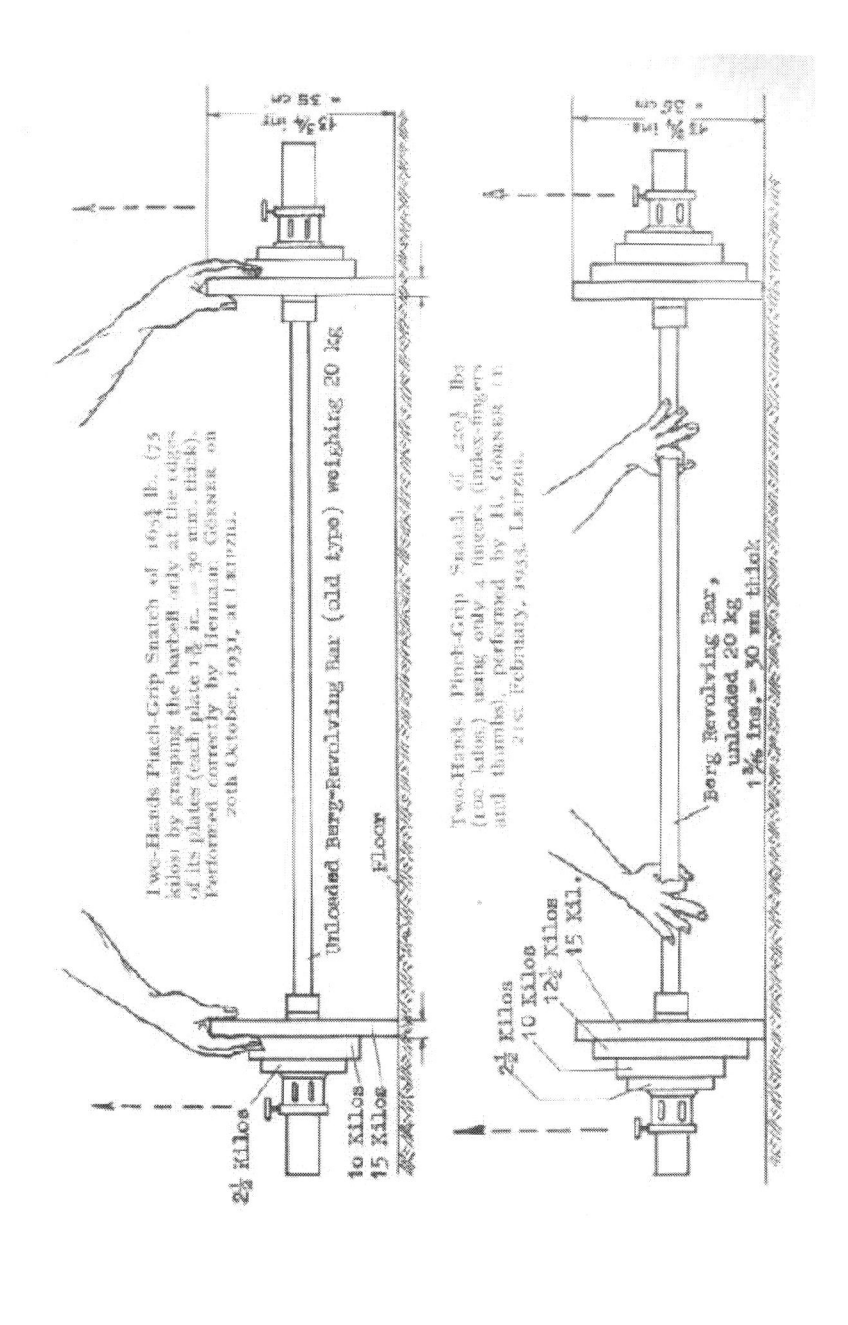

Two-Hands Pinch-Grip Snatch of 165¼ lb. (75 kilos) by grasping the barbell only at the edge of its plates (each plate 1⅛ in. = 30 mm. thick). Performed correctly by Hermann GÖRNER on 20th October, 1933, at LEIPZIG.

Unloaded Berg-Revolving Bar (old type) weighing 20 kg

Floor

2½ Kilos
10 Kilos
15 Kilos

Two-Hands Pinch-Grip Snatch of 220¼ lb. (100 kilos), using only 4 fingers (index-fingers and thumbs), performed by H. GÖRNER on 21st February, 1933, LEIPZIG.

Berg Revolving Bar, unloaded 20 kg 1¾ ins. = 30 mm thick

2½ Kilos
10 Kilos
12½ Kilos
15 Kil.

In his book, published in 1926 and entitled *The Key to Might and Muscle*, Jowett illustrated a chapter with the posed picture of Görner and Hermann's great friend, Tromp van Diggelen of South Africa, and uses the following remark:

> "Tromp van Diggelen introducing Hermann Görner, the greatest man of might and muscle of all times; greater than Cyr, Apollon, or Saxon. He has brought forward with him a new era in which the clean cut type is combined with incredible strength. 6 ft. 1 in. and 245 lb. – HE HAS POWER WITHOUT LIMIT!"

Tromp van Diggelen of Capetown, South Africa, who is the most knowledgeable authority of that country in every branch of physical culture and a man I felt honoured to meet in Leipzig in 1934. He has been a close crony of Hermann Görner since 1908 and they have been the strongest of friends over these many years.

Van Diggelen was the first man to make known to the English-speaking public that a true superman lived among them. In 1926, 3rd April to be exact, Tromp van Diggelen, in a striking article in the English magazine, *Health and Strength*, aroused the Physical Culture World, with the words,

> "Is there a stronger man in the world than Hermann Görner?"

In the *Cape Times* the same author penned the following statements,

> "I have personally known most of the world's recognized Strong Men and many people will remember that in 1909 I introduced Maxick, the most phenomenal Strong Man for his weight the world had ever known, to the British public in London, but never have I known a man to possess the colossal strength that Görner is gifted with".

Bob Hoffman of York, U.S.A. The founder of the famous York

EDGAR MÜLLER

Barbell Club, trainer of more World's Champions and Olympic Champions than any other man. Editor and publisher of *Strength and Health* magazine, and himself a physical giant and one of the world's Strong Men, wrote in one of his many books,

> "Görner is a contender for the title 'Strongest Man of all Time'".

Henry Graf of Bern, Switzerland, former World's Feather Weight Champion, writing in *Athletik* for 26th February, 1931, wrote,

> "Hermann Görner, a biceps colossus of the largest type, performing with Pagel's circus and gaining overwhelming favour in South Africa, has, in carrying and lifting heavy weights, no opponents at the present time in the world. Where rugged primitive strength is concerned, he has no equal. In considering Charles Rigolout as the present World's Champion Weight Lifter, we must certainly regard Görner as the World's Strongest Man".

Professor Ferdinand Hueppe of Dresden and formerly of the University of Prague, one of the greatest European authorities on hygiene and physical culture, in addition to being an anthropometrist, said as follows,

> "I have had the honour of interviewing and inspecting the feats of Hermann Görner, the world's record holder and Strong Man of Leipzig. I, personally, on 11th July, 1920, witnessed his Clean and Jerk with barbell of 390 ¼ lb. On 20th July, I watched him do a right-hand dead lift with a sandstone block lifted between his legs weighing 734 ½ lb., standing fully erect with this prodigious burden. To-day (this was written on 25th July, 1920) he raised in the shape of four kettleweights in the Two Hands 'Anyhow' a weight of no less than 430 lb. Truly a stupendous feat beyond the ability of any other athlete".

Hugo Rosch, champion athlete and wrestler of Saxony, in an

article written in a German magazine made the following assertion,

> "Hermann Görner, following his quite phenomenal feats of recent times, such as his 'carrying on back' performances, as observed by myself, leaves one with the impression that he does not know his own strength – his feats are so colossal that they have to be seen to be believed".

Gordon Venables, former Managing Editor of Bob Hoffman's magazine, *Strength and Health*, writing in the book *Mighty Men of Old*, had this to say about Hermann Görner,

> "Known to Iron Men as the 'Monarch of Strength' was Hermann Görner, giant South African Dutchman. He stood 6 ft. 1 in. tall, weighed 245 lb. his expanded chest was 52 ½ in., biceps 18 ¼ in., forearm 16 in. and thighs 27 in. He holds the world record in the One-hand Dead Lift with 602 lb. He has jerked 397 lb. to arms length from behind the neck, continentalled 440 lb. to his chest and jerked 264 lb. overhead with one hand. He once performed a stunt that lifters never cease to wonder at, a snatch of 231 lb. with the hands crossed. On the stage, one of his famous feats was the supporting of a trestle bridge over which an automobile with five passengers was driven. The total weight was 5,500 lb."

In *Muscle Power* magazine for November, 1946 an article entitled "What is a good Build?" by Jack Reid, had the following to say about Hermann Görner,

> "Taking my choice among Heavyweights, I might say that the photos of Görner give me an impression of the presence of great force. To my mind this athlete combines a strength which is exceedingly rare and one which is not encumbered by the gross bulk of the 'Cyr' type or that peculiar to the Austrian lifters round the early 1900's. Görner, furthermore, combines size with height, which eliminates the 'squatty' look that a man of short stature and equal bulk might bear".

EDGAR MÜLLER

W.A. Pullum of London, known popularly as the 'Wizard of the Weight Lifting World', Coach to the English Olympic Weight Lifting Team of 1948, one of Britain's leading trainers and coaches, former World's Champion and record holder introduced Hermann Görner to a dazzled British public in 1927 in the following terms,

"The strongest of all the world's strongest men".
On another occasion,
"Hercules comes back to Earth".

His faithful recountings of the amazing performances he had witnessed of Görner became a special feature of the English *Health and Strength* magazine at that time.

Otto Buettner of Leipzig, well-known sports' writer, devoted five full pages in a glowing tribute to the world's first wonderman of strength, in a newspaper which made a feature of the enthralling life of Görner.

John E. Dawe, BAWLA referee, writer, reporter and practical exponent of the Strength cult, an intimate of most of the world's strongest men and a constant visitor to Hermann Görner in Germany, made the following comment in *Strength and Health*, issue July, 1949,

"Although he (Görner) is now 58, he does not look his age and could take off 10 years. He is quite massive – his neck, arms and shoulders are huge and show no sign of shrinkage".

Ray van Cleef, popular Associate Editor of *Strength and Health*, known as the 'Ambassador of Strength', never tires of writing of the legendary might of Görner. During the year 1949, Ray wrote on many occasions articles relating to the past feats of Hermann Görner, which were published in *Strength and Health* magazine.

Ian "Mac" Batchelor, gigantic American strongman, famous wrist-wrestling champion and notable sports writer, had the following to say about Hermann Görner in the June, 1950, issue of *Muscle Power*:

"Hermann Görner, another immense physique! What a back! Probably the greatest dead-lifter of all time, huge proportions, a dynamo of power. His arms and legs exerted gigantic impulse due to his back strength surpassing that of his limbs in a vast degree."

Leo Gaudreau, noted athlete and one of America's leading authorities on famous Strong Men, made the following comment in an article entitled "The Mighty Görner" in *Your Physique* magazine for July 1950 : –

"The great Hermann Görner, considered by many as being the strongest man who ever lived!"

It is not possible to include in this book many other appreciations of Görner by other well-known authorities, but by the foregoing extracts readers will be able to judge for themselves the esteem held for this King among Strongmen.

For completing this summary of the estimation of the World of Strength on the ability and prowess of Hermann Görner, it may be mentioned that he was selected as an Honorary Member by the following Clubs and Associations:

1. Kraftsportverein "Atlas", Leipzig.
2. Vereinigung "Die Alten Leipziger Athleten" (DALA).
3. American Continental Weightlifters' Association.
4. Hermann Görner Sport Club, Leipzig.
5. Turn and Sportverein "1867" Leipzig.
6. Turn and Sportverein, Klein Heidorn.

This, then, is the story of Hermann Görner. The story of a man the like of whom the world may never see again: the story of the one man whose strength has long been a by-word in the World of Strength, but whose exact feats and performances have never been revealed until now. In setting forth this factual recital of the life and feats of this King among Strong Men, it is the earnest hope of the Author that it may inspire others to follow in the footsteps of the subject of this book – the incomparable Hermann Görner.

For more old time classics of strength, visit:

StrongmanBooks.com

Sign up on the website for a free gift and updates about new books added regularly.

Titles Available About and From All These Authors:

Arthur Saxon	William Blaikie
Bob Hoffman	Farmer Burns
Maxick	Monte Saldo
Eugen Sandow	Lionel Strongfort
George F. Jowett	Antone Matysek
Otto Arco	Harry Paschall
George Hackenschmidt	Louis Cyr
Thomas Inch	Alois Swoboda
Edward Aston	William Pullum
Bernarr MacFadden	Joe Bonomo
Earle Liederman	Siegmund Breitbart
Alan Calvert	Mighty Apollon
Alexander Zass	And Many More

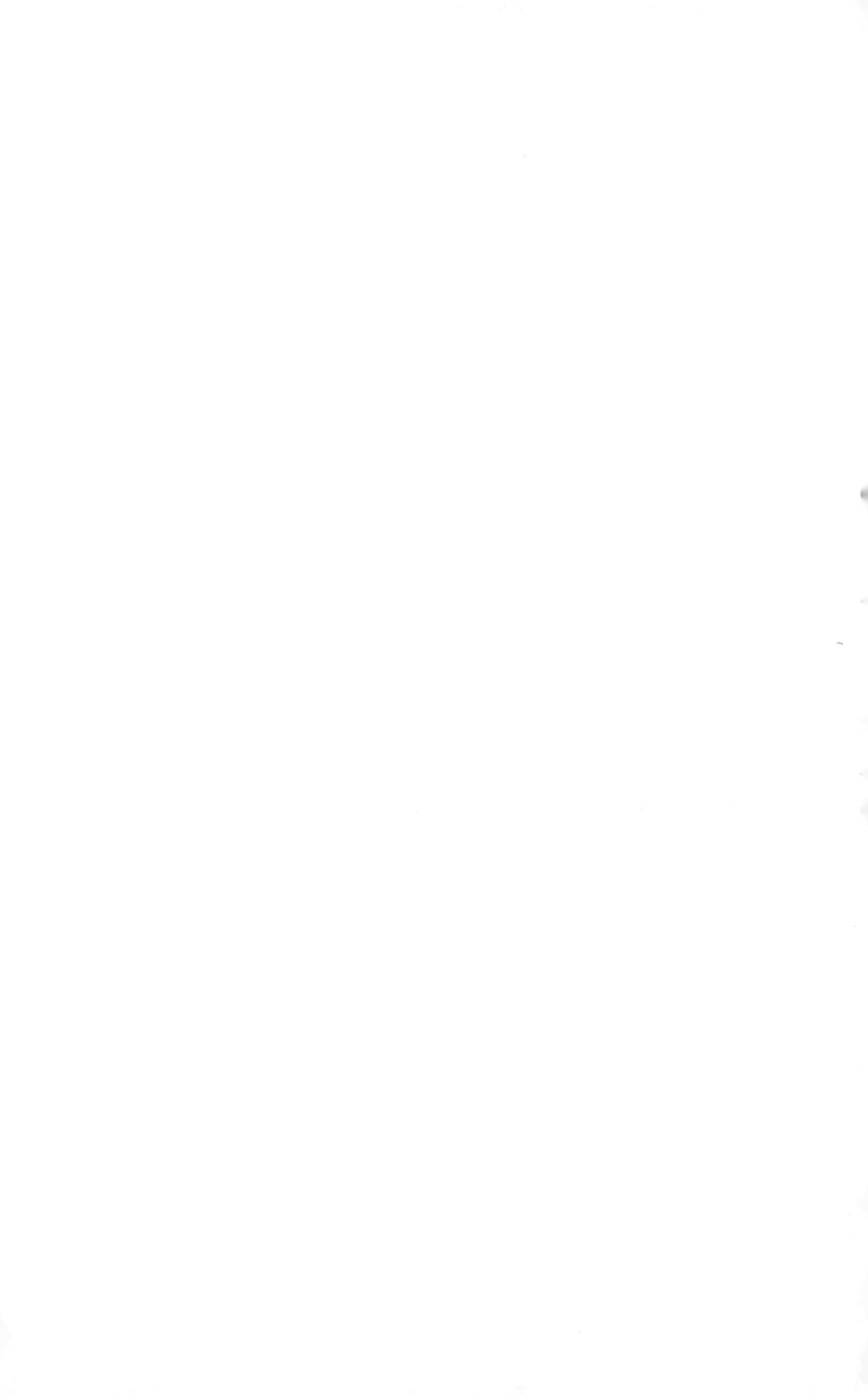

Printed in Great Britain
by Amazon.co.uk, Ltd.,
Marston Gate.